Overcoming Common Problems Series

For a full list of titles please contact
Sheldon Press, Marylebone Road, London NW1 4DU

Antioxidants
DR ROBERT YOUNGSON

The Assertiveness Workbook
JOANNA GUTMANN

Beating the Comfort Trap
DR WINDY DRYDEN AND JACK
GORDON

Body Language
ALLAN PEASE

Body Language in Relationships
DAVID COHEN

Calm Down
DR PAUL HAUCK

Cancer – A Family Affair
NEVILLE SHONE

The Cancer Guide for Men
HELEN BEARE AND NEIL PRIDDY

The Candida Diet Book
KAREN BRODY

Caring for Your Elderly Parent
JULIA BURTON-JONES

Cider Vinegar
MARGARET HILLS

Comfort for Depression
JANET HORWOOD

Considering Adoption?
SARAH BIGGS

Coping Successfully with Hay Fever
DR ROBERT YOUNGSON

Coping Successfully with Pain
NEVILLE SHONE

Coping Successfully with Panic Attacks
SHIRLEY TRICKETT

Coping Successfully with PMS
KAREN EVENNETT

Coping Successfully with Prostate Problems
ROSY REYNOLDS

Coping Successfully with RSI
MAGGIE BLACK AND PENNY GRAY

Coping Successfully with Your Hiatus Hernia
DR TOM SMITH

Coping Successfully with Your Irritable Bladder
DR JENNIFER HUNT

Coping Successfully with Your Irritable Bowel
ROSEMARY NICOL

Coping When Your Child Has Special Needs
SUZANNE ASKHAM

Coping with Anxiety and Depression
SHIRLEY TRICKETT

Coping with Blushing
DR ROBERT EDELMANN

Coping with Bronchitis and Emphysema
DR TOM SMITH

Coping with Candida
SHIRLEY TRICKETT

Coping with Chronic Fatigue
TRUDIE CHALDER

Coping with Coeliac Disease
KAREN BRODY

Coping with Cystitis
CAROLINE CLAYTON

Coping with Depression and Elation
DR PATRICK McKEON

Coping with Eczema
DR ROBERT YOUNGSON

Coping with Endometriosis
JO MEARS

Coping with Epilepsy
FIONA MARSHALL AND
DR PAMELA CRAWFORD

Coping with Fibroids
MARY-CLAIRE MASON

Coping with Gallstones
DR JOAN GOMEZ

Coping with Headaches and Migraine
SHIRLEY TRICKETT

Coping with a Hernia
DR DAVID DELVIN

Coping with Psoriasis
PROFESSOR RONALD MARKS

Coping with Rheumatism and Arthritis
DR ROBERT YOUNGSON

Coping with Stammering
TRUDY STEWART AND JACKIE
TURNBULL

Coping with Stomach Ulcers
DR TOM SMITH

Overcoming Common Problems Series

Overcoming Common Problems Series

Overcoming Common Problems

How to Lose Weight
Without Dieting

Mark Barker

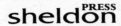
sheldon PRESS

Published in Great Britain in 2001 by
Sheldon Press
SPCK, Holy Trinity Church
Marylebone Road
London NW1 4DU

British Library Cataloguing-in-Publication Data

A catalogue for this book is available from the British Library

ISBN 0–85969–860–2

Typeset by Deltatype Limited, Birkenhead, Merseyside
Printed in Great Britain by
Biddles Ltd, www.biddles.co.uk

Contents

This book is dedicated to my mother who always encouraged me, to my father whose love of learning helped open my mind, and to all my clients who taught me so much.

Slimming with Psychology

Programme objectives

This ten-week programme is designed to enable you to:

- Lose weight steadily and stabilize at a weight at which you feel comfortable (without dieting).
- Enjoy your food, without the love/hate swings.
- Eat to live, rather than live to eat.
- Eat only when hungry.
- Say goodbye to binges.
- Be more confident and happy.
- Be better able to cope with emotions.
- Have more fulfilling relationships.
- Stop feeling guilty.
- Expand your horizons in life and be a success.

What does the programme consist of?

The programme consists of four parts:

Part 1: Introduction and guidelines

The first section clarifies your suitability for the programme and discusses the ineffectiveness of dieting. Clear guidelines are given to help you make the programme work.

Part 2: Understanding the underlying causes of your weight/eating problem

This section focuses on the emotional and psychological factors that can powerfully affect eating habits. Your own conditioning will be covered in some detail so that you will be able to explore the underlying cause of your eating problems.

Part 3: The psychological and practical solutions

The third section shows you how to take more control of your life using assertiveness, habit change and the ability to satisfy your emotional needs. You will decide what changes you need to make in your attitudes and behaviour in order to solve your eating problems.

Part 4: Action plan

This is the time for action. You will know what you have to do, why you have to do it and how to put your plan into action. This fourth section consists of a ten-week plan with step-by-step measures which will guarantee success.

PART 1
Introduction and Guidelines

Introduction

This is no ordinary weight-loss programme. There is not a single diet or exercise schedule. There is no need for bulking agents or appetite-suppressing drugs. In order to help you understand how I discovered the secrets of permanent weight control, let me take you back a few years.

In 1982, having had appropriate training, I began practising as a private psychotherapist and hypnotherapist. People came with problems as diverse as nailbiting and fear of flying. But by far the most common problem was that of weight control, and it was mainly women who were wanting help.

On average, I was being consulted by ten women per week with some form of eating problem. Over five years, this resulted in about 2,500 therapy sessions that involved women and food.

Some of my clients wanted to lose just one stone, others wanted to shed four, five or even more. Some ate a little too much, others binged themselves. Indeed, some were not overweight at all, but food or body image was still ruling their lives. Some were teenagers, others pensioners.

Through this diversity there began to emerge a common thread running through the lives of these clients – and it had nothing directly to do with food. It was this discovery that made me understand why so many women asked me questions such as:

'Why can't I stick to a diet?'
'Why do I feel so guilty?'
'After dieting so hard, why do I put the weight back on?'
'Why do I turn to food when I'm lonely, angry or depressed?'
'I know what foods I should eat, but why do I like all the wrong foods?'
'I think about food all the time; how can I break free of these thoughts?'

When I began to help clients find answers to these sort of questions I was amazed at how solutions to their eating problems became crystal clear. In a matter of weeks, clients began changing habits that had been with them for years.

In this programme I have distilled what went on in those hundreds of therapy sessions, seeking the recurring themes, and have added the latest psychological techniques to enable you to solve your weight/eating problem – *permanently.*

I want you to share in the success and freedom that the vast majority of clients gained from their sessions. Their success took between five and ten weeks, consisting of one hourly session per week with me followed by the vital factor of making changes themselves in their everyday life.

This programme consists of a ten-week plan of action. It has been designed from the start as a self-help programme, but if you have a good friend who would like to go through the programme at the same time, it may be valuable for you both to spend time together discussing each other's progress, problems and ideas.

NOTE: I am not claiming my insights into eating problems are unique; other therapists and psychologists have now come to similar conclusions. Indeed, these back up my findings and give me confidence in the basic principles on which this programme is based. What I do claim are unique are *the solutions offered to the problem.* While researching material that had already been published I found time and time again an over-emphasis on analysing the problem, rather than *concentrating on the solutions.* You want solutions. This programme has them for you to find.

Are you suitable for this programme?

Although most of my clients were overweight and wanted to lose weight, some clients were at a satisfactory weight but struggling to stay there. The methods in this programme worked for both groups. That is why I talk not just about weight problems but also about weight/eating problems.

Two extreme eating disorders are anorexia (self-starvation) and bulimia (self-starvation with periods of bingeing and self-induced vomiting). Although these two serious problems have different symptoms, they share many of the same causes. I would recommend professional one-to-one help for these extreme eating disorders, but even for these much help may be found in the following pages.

To test your suitability for this programme, answer the following questions:

1 Have you tried several types of diet?
2 Have most or all of these diets failed sooner or later?
3 Do you sometimes dislike yourself?
4 Is food on your mind a great deal of the time?
5 Do you eat when not hungry?
6 Is your self-confidence shaky?
7 Do you often eat for comfort?
8 Do you ever go on binges?
9 Do your relationships with other adults leave much room for improvement?
10 Do you feel that your life is out of your control?

If you answered 'yes' to five or more then you are *very* suitable for this programme. Two to four 'yes' responses means that you are *satisfactorily* suitable. A 'yes' score of less than two means that you should try a different approach to solving your problem.

The magic pill

Some clients, on their first session, would say, 'Oh, just hypnotize me and tell me not to eat.' This is an understandable request bearing in mind that we live in a society where the 'magic pill' is offered so freely. A pill for depression, a pill for nerves, a pill for vitamins, a pill for appetite suppression. Just read the adverts: 'Vibrate those flabby inches away', 'New wonder cardboard which prevents calories being absorbed' or 'Revolutionary electronic calorie counter'. How many times have you seen: 'This new diet really works'?

All these products have three things in common:

1 They offer to do all the work for you (implying that it is easy).
2 They are not selective (suggesting that everyone has the same needs).
3 Their results are at best only temporary (when you stop taking the 'magic pill' the original problem rears its ugly head – often with renewed vigour).

Research shows that 97 per cent of slimmers
regain the weight they worked so hard to lose

I rejected the magic pill solution because it simply does not work. So I did not wave the hypnotic magic wand. (Most hypnosis tapes on the market are only providing short-term results. However, when used in conjunction with this programme a hypnotic tape could be beneficial.)

I believe that you do have the ability to understand and solve your problems, initially with my help along the way. I believe that *you* are a wonderful, unique human being and I regret that I cannot work with you face to face. There are things that I could learn from you and I hope you will write to me about how you have progressed with the programme. I would also welcome any suggestions for improving material presented to you here. This programme could not have been written without the feedback from my clients.

I also believe that you have a vast reservoir of untapped potential, waiting to be used. I cannot be sure, but I would guess that you are fed up with promises of wonder cures and are searching for a deeper, long-lasting solution.

How to use this book

This book is a *workbook*. A workbook helps you to understand and solve your problems as you go along and it requires input from you.

A workbook makes you involved and interested because you are the central character. Your ideas and insights should be written down in the book, building up your case history, with you becoming your own therapist, with my guidance.

When you have completed the programme and refer back to this workbook, you may well be surprised about how much you have changed in a relatively short space of time.

A workbook requires you to expend some effort, and this is vitally important. *Change needs effort.* Most ordinary books are just read through, and however brilliant the ideas are they rarely make a deep and long-lasting impact. Think about the differences between watching a holiday programme on television and actually going on a holiday yourself. The TV experience finishes at the end of the programme, but the real holiday lasts in your memory, perhaps for ever.

I assure you the effort required in this programme is a fraction of the effort you have already spent on dieting, and a fraction of the cost!

Effort does not mean hard work. If you are interested and motivated, effort is natural and gives you a sense of achievement.

The biggest obstacles to your success are probably your lack of motivation and your fear of failure

To help motivation, ask yourself, 'Do I want to live with my weight/eating problem for the next year . . . the next five years . . . the rest of my life . . . ?'

Some fears are healthy, such as the fear which we would feel if we were to walk very close to the edge of a cliff on a windy day. This fear protects us from genuine danger. However, most people's fears are based on imagined dangers. These imagined dangers are caused by expecting that the worst will happen. So, if you suffer from fear of failure, try the following exercise:

Imagine that you are really expecting this programme to work for you

Drum the positive expectancy into your mind, 'I want this to work and it will work, it will work, it will work . . .' Now take a deep breath and say out loud in a firm, positive voice, 'I am going to make this work and it will work.' Do you sound convincing? Perhaps not totally at first, but as you work through the programme your confidence will grow.

PROGRAMME GUIDELINES

Before you launch into the programme I would like you to understand what I'm going to ask you to do.

Guideline 1: Stop dieting

Let us start with defining what we mean by dieting, because the word 'diet' has two meanings. If a person is described as 'having a healthy diet' that describes their permanent way of eating. However, if somebody is 'on a diet' that describes a temporary way of eating in order to lose weight. Some slimming diets are much better than others, but they are all temporary and have many powerful emotions attached to them, which can lead to dieting becoming compulsive.

Compulsive dieting is the reverse of compulsive eating. One breeds the other. They become a vicious circle. You can break the destructive circle at the dieting stage by understanding the reasons why dieting is bad news.

1 *Diets do not work.* No diet you have ever been on has worked permanently, otherwise you would not be starting this programme. Perhaps a diet has worked for a while – but that is not good enough.

2 *Diets fail – so try something different.*

3 *Diets make you eat more.* Dieting creates a feeling of missing out and suffering. Have you ever finished a diet and then eaten lots of 'naughties' to make up for the deprivation?

4 *Diets create guilt.* Have you ever 'cheated' while dieting only to have your treat ruined by guilt?

5 *Dieting makes an enemy of food.* We need food to live; we have to eat. But dieting labels certain foods 'bad' and others 'good'. We often like to eat the 'bad' foods. It therefore develops into a love/hate relationship with food, whereas food should give us pure pleasure, undiminished by guilt.

6 *Dieting makes you hungry.* Often the foods or meal-substitute drinks make you hungry and the constant thought about food triggers hunger pangs sooner still. If you stay hungry you suffer, if you succumb you feel guilty. You cannot win.

7 *Diets make you obsessed with food and/or calories.* The more restricted you are, the more your mind will become preoccupied with food and eating. These unwanted thoughts can start dominating your life. Dieters often really do live to diet. Extreme eating disorders can then take hold.

8 *Dieting makes you lose touch with your bodily needs.* By ignoring natural body signals which tell you when you should eat, you start fighting your body signals rather than learning how to interpret them, as every wild animal does instinctively. This makes it harder to re-establish a natural, healthy eating pattern.

9 *Dieting makes you feel a failure.* The more times a diet has failed, the more likely you are to blame yourself and feel a sense of shame.

10 *Diets make you confused.* Who should you believe? The high-protein supporters, the high-fibre lobby, the lean-meat people, the grape fans . . . ?

11 *Dieting can make you fat.* A very low calorie diet will reduce not only fat, but also lean tissue (muscle). Fine if you keep at that weight, but very few do. When the old eating habits return the fat may go back on faster than the lean tissue. So, if you started at 10 st, lost 2 st rapidly, then just as quickly went back up to 10 st, the proportion of body fat may have increased.

It has also been proved that low calorie diets reduce your metabolic rate. Your body tries to conserve the meagre rations it is given. This means calories are burned up more slowly, making weight even more difficult to lose!

How depressing!   *Are you convinced?*

NOTE: You may find it difficult to stop dieting. If the thought of not dieting is uncomfortable, you may be compulsive about dieting. Some people feel they deserve to suffer for being so out of control, fat or greedy. There may be a fear about rapid weight gain when dieting ends.

Eleven reasons have just been given for *not* dieting. How many reasons can you think of *for* dieting? The compulsive dieter may have to go through a gradual process of letting go of the need to diet. The first step is to acknowledge the strong case against dieting, and to realize that your world will not fall apart when you stop dieting.

Conflicting messages

The glossy adverts in women's magazines send out a powerful repetitive message encouraging diets and diet foods.

However, many of the feature articles in the same magazines, written by eating therapists and psychologists, are telling a different story. These features talk about, 'How fear can make you fat', 'Fat – the stress factor', or 'Do you eat for comfort?' Most of these features contain good ideas, but fail to make a lasting impact because they are so very short. They can only talk generally and skim the surface. This programme encompasses many of the good ideas you probably have already read in these articles and takes them much further and deeper.

Guideline 2: Eat the food you like

This second guideline may seem strange, even frightening. Suppose you like chocolate and chips. How can eating these foods help you lose weight? The reasoning goes like this:

7

By having 'thou shalt not' attached to certain foods you like, you suffer because you do not allow yourself to eat them. This deprivation makes you crave them all the more. When you finally give way to these cravings it is inevitable that you will feel guilty. The guilt leads to renewed dieting and the vicious circle is complete.

When you stop dieting and begin to solve the underlying causes of your eating problem, you will relearn to listen to the signals that your body is sending. You will be able to hear your body saying, 'I only want one chocolate' without your mind intervening and saying much louder, 'I want the whole box.' Your body will say, 'Eat that nutritious salad, not that fattening stodge or that empty sugar.' So you will lose weight by eating less of the fattening foods and more of the naturally slimming foods. You will be eating for your physical needs, not your emotional needs.

Eventually you will automatically choose those foods which are healthy and your whole way of eating will improve as you begin to care for your body rather than abuse it. Your desire will be not just to be slim, but to be slim and healthy.

Guideline 3: Don't go hungry

Hunger is another form of suffering. Skipping meals and going hungry, like the other ways of suffering with food, leads to food being constantly on the mind.

There is a very important law:

The harder you try not to think of something,
the more often it will be on your mind

Example: try *not* to think of a double-decker bus floating in the air ... What just came into your mind?

The consequence of this law is that it is virtually impossible to blot out food from your mind when you are hungry. This programme will help you eat when you are hungry and not eat when you are not hungry. After all, your body has been designed that way over millions of years!

Guideline 4: Exercise if you enjoy it

If you enjoy exercise you are responding to the natural signals of your body. That's great. Exercise can make you feel physically and mentally good. I thoroughly recommend it. It may be just choosing to walk somewhere rather than going in a vehicle. In the wild, animals eat when hungry, drink when thirsty and exercise as a natural part of their lives. You never see a fat wild animal, only fat pets that have been given a similar lifestyle to their human owners.

If you don't enjoy exercise, don't force it – don't suffer. When you relearn to respond to your body signals, exercise will become an enjoyable part of everyday life.

CAUTION: As with dieting, exercising has now become big business. The media pressurize us to be fit. Lycra-clad celebrities are on countless videos. Women such as Jane Fonda have now extended the age range in which you 'should' be seen to be going to keep-fit classes in expensive designer sports wear. The pressure is on right up to and beyond middle age.

Until recently the price you have to pay for an 'ideal' body has been kept a secret. After 23 years of suffering, Jane Fonda has courageously spoken out:

> Society says we have to be thin, and while most of us don't have much control of our lives, we can control our weight, either by starving to death or by eating all we want and not showing the effects . . . I loved to eat but I wanted to be wonderfully thin. It didn't take long for me to become a serious bulimic – bingeing and purging 15 to 20 times a day! . . . bulimia was my secret 'vice'. No one was supposed to find out about it, and because I was supposed to be so strong and perfect, I couldn't admit to myself that I had a weakness and a serious disease.

Ex Spice Girl Geri Halliwell has recently been reported to have been suffering from bulimia for some time. I'm sure many of the glamorous female icons have a really difficult time with their eating and weight.

Uma Thurman, star of *Pulp Fiction*, and *Dangerous Liaisons*, has confessed to having a psychological problem about her weight. She is convinced she is overweight. 'I see myself as fat,' she said.

So don't be fooled by the perfect image. There is often suffering lying behind the perfect façade. Chasing illusions is the recipe for unhappiness

Guideline 5: Do not use slimming tablets or bulking agents

These are the literal 'magic pills' which I discussed earlier. At best, they produce only temporary weight loss. At worst, they aggravate the eating problems and may have damaging side-effects. They separate you further from your body signals.

Guideline 6: Work through the programme step by step

It is impossible to run before you can walk. This programme has been designed so that you can succeed over a ten-week period, step by step. The path to success consists of several shorter stages which are all achievable. This is the case when learning anything new, from learning to type to learning to play the piano. The confidence you gain as you master stage after stage will grow into a snowball of positive attitudes. The new feelings of success will crush the old feelings of failure.

Guideline 7: If you suspect you have a physical problem consult your doctor

This programme is for those with emotional and psychological eating problems, who make up the largest group of those with eating disorders. However, if you suspect that you do have a physical problem, please consult your doctor before starting the programme.

GUIDELINE SUMMARY

1 Do not diet.
2 Eat the food you like.
3 Don't go hungry.
4 Exercise if you enjoy it.
5 No 'magic pills'.
6 Work through step by step.
7 If you suspect a physical problem consult your doctor.

You are not expected to follow all these guidelines perfectly at first, but introduce them when you feel ready. Remember, these guidelines are not just for the ten-week programme, but for life.

Now you are ready to move on to Part 2 of the programme.

PART 2

Understanding the Causes of Your Eating Problem

Introduction

There are two main reasons why people find it difficult to lose weight permanently. The first reason is poor eating and lifestyle habits that are difficult to change. The second is the existence of an underlying psychological need that drives the eating. Many people will have both reasons operating at the same time. This explains why millions of people struggle so hard with weight loss. In Part 2 you will discover whether you have poor eating habits, an unresolved psychological need, or both. At this stage keep an open mind. Work through both sections and then decide at the end of Part 2 what is the cause of your eating problems.

POOR EATING HABITS

Eating habits, like all habits, are not only in the mind, but are 'wired' into our brains and bodies. It is important to understand the nature of habits because then you will better appreciate the methods that I will give you to break the old habits and create new healthy ones. Let us look deeper into habitual behaviour.

Neuro-mental association

I would like to introduce you to a term that I have coined to help understand habits: neuro-mental association (NMA).

- Neuro refers to neurology and the connections in the nervous system.
- Mental refers to thoughts, beliefs and emotions.
- Association is the meaning that the neuro-mental functions put on external events.

An example will help you understand the theory of NMA. If you are

11

driving and see a person ahead step on to a zebra crossing you will, almost certainly, automatically move your right foot and brake. You don't have to think, you just act. Your eye sees an image and that image triggers an automatic response from your body. This is a strong NMA for most of us living in the UK. In some other countries this NMA is absent (beware, pedestrians!). In the UK we have been conditioned to link serious repercussions with not respecting zebra crossings.

This NMA was started when you were a child and your parents would teach you to cross the road at the black and white stripes. As a passenger, you then observed the driver stopping for people to cross. Then, when you were learning to drive, the instructor reminded you to be careful every time a pedestrian crossing was approached and to be prepared to brake. If you performed correctly you received praise; if you did not prepare to brake you would suffer a severe reprimand. This repetition created pathways in your brain. Also, you believed that it was the right thing to do, so you did not resist the instructions you were given. You saw other drivers stopping when pedestrians put a foot on the crossing, so your behaviour was in line with your peer group.

Eventually, your nervous system was conditioned by praise and reprimand to automatically act a certain way (neuro). Your beliefs supported your actions and the emotion of fear of knocking someone down was strong (mental). Seeing the pedestrian begin to step meant that they were about to cross (association).

The theory of neuro-mental association helps us understand the complex and interactive way habits are formed. Your eating habits have also been created by a mixture of different forces that have reinforced each other. Being social animals, many of our habits are dependent on the society in which we live, including our eating habits. For example, the UK has the highest obesity rate in Europe. If you compare the length of our supermarket shelves of biscuits, crisps and sugary drinks with those in other countries, you get an idea of how ingrained poor eating habits are in the UK. We in the UK have developed a convenience food culture. Unfortunately, most convenience foods are high in fat and sugar and other highly processed ingredients, that give us calories but precious little real nourishment. So you have to decide not to follow the crowd and buy the poor food that is put in front of you in the supermarkets or the fast food take-aways. There is some great healthy food in supermarkets as well, but you have to hunt it out, hidden among the highly advertised processed foods. Your excessive weight could be caused by simply being brought up in a country like the UK or the USA where the food available is generally of a high calorie, low nutritional nature.

Eating a certain way is a cultural habit. The Scots and the Northern Irish have the highest heart-related deaths in the world. The cause is the food eaten. The great Scottish breakfast of porridge (one of the healthiest foods) turned into the fry-up. There is also a huge difference in the food you eat depending on the socio-economic group you grew up in. The UK is still a class-divided society in which it is very difficult for some people even to access good wholesome foods. While the middle classes embrace brown bread, organic fruit and vegetables from fashionable shops, many people living in large housing estates have only one shop, which does not sell fresh fruit or vegetables at all, but has every fatty potato snack you can imagine. So your current weight problems could be mainly because of the foods you have grown up with: a cultural eating habit.

There is one question that will tell you if your eating problem is caused by simple habit alone:

Do your emotions affect what you eat?

If the answer is an unconditional 'no', then the section in Part 3 on changing habits may be enough to help you lose weight permanently. Even if your answer is 'no', I recommend continuing through the rest of Part 2 to be absolutely sure that there are no other causes that you are unaware of.

The vast majority of people will answer 'yes' to the above question. Of course, the answers will vary from 'yes, sometimes' to 'yes, completely and utterly'.

You almost certainly do not know the real cause of your eating problem. If you did, then you probably would have solved it by now. You may know some of the things that make it worse – perhaps an argument or a bout of depression – but *why* do you turn to food? Just saying that it's comfort eating doesn't really tell us much, it is just a description.

In this section I hope that you will discover the real underlying cause of your eating problem. The root cause may be a complete surprise to you. You may even find it difficult to believe at first. But when you have found it and accepted it, many puzzling things that you do will suddenly make sense – not least your battle with food.

In Part 2 you will find several different causes of eating problems. I have included a wide range of possible causes to cater for the many different people using this programme. Perhaps only one is relevant to you. That is all you are looking for – your causal factor. Once found, the solution will become clear and you will begin, in Parts 3 and 4, to make changes that will enhance your life, not just solve your eating problem.

One client said, 'It's like starting the rest of my life with the slate clean.'

SYMPTOMS AND CAUSES

The reason why I did not use simple 'you will eat less' hypnosis on clients who had a history of eating problems is because it would have worked only on the symptom and not on the underlying cause. I might have had a happy client for two or three weeks, but when the old eating habits returned it would be, 'That hypnotherapy is no good – it doesn't last.' It would be like trying to get rid of a dandelion by just removing the leaves. If you have ever tried this you will know that more leaves appear in a couple of weeks.

Consider the case of a child who begins to be bullied at school and suddenly starts scoring lower marks in tests. A teacher may simply tell the child off and give her extra homework. However, a good teacher would want to find out why the change in results has occurred. The good teacher would ask the child questions and gather information to discover the cause of the decline. Then the teacher would try to help the child solve the bullying problem. In this case the *cause* is the bullying and the *symptom* is the lower marks.

The central principle of this programme is that your eating/weight problem may be a symptom of an underlying cause. Whenever we suffer unpleasant symptoms we are motivated to find the cause. A sharp stabbing pain in the foot while walking will not be endured for many steps. Soon the shoe is off and the thorn is found and removed. When we feel a tickle, we waste no time in flicking the fly away. This can be summarized by two laws of causes and symptoms:

1 We seek the causes of symptoms.
2 When the cause is found, we desire to remove it.

However, as I earlier suggested, most people with eating problems have been unable to find the real cause, let alone remove it. This leads us to the third law:

3 When we suffer from a symptom and can't find the cause, we feel helpless, vulnerable, confused and probably anxious.

Wouldn't you feel like this if you had a stabbing pain in your foot, but couldn't find the thorn? Because of this third law, it is in the interest of those earning millions of pounds selling diet books, diet foods and all the other 'magic pills' to keep their customers in the dark. As long as we feel helpless and worried we will try anything, even though we know deep down this is not the real answer. It is said that knowledge is power. Later in the programme that power will be returned to its rightful owner – *you*.

The peeling wallpaper example

The cause–symptom principle is so important. Let's consider another example:

Imagine that, unknown to you, a slate has slipped off the roof of your house. But all you notice is that the wallpaper is coming away from your bedroom wall. What do you do?

Well, Option 1 would be to do nothing and live with it. But how would you feel every time you noticed it? Would it nag away at you? Option 2 would be to paste it back up – after all, it would look all right for a while. Option 3 would be to go outside and see if any damp is coming through the roof. This last option involves effort and acceptance that there may be more effort ahead if any repairs are needed.

Option 1 is the ostrich-like 'head in the sand' approach: try to ignore it and hope it will go away. Experience shows that this doesn't work very often and could even make the problem worse. In this case the whole ceiling could come down if the problem is ignored.

Option 2 is the 'sweeping the problem under the carpet' method. Things can appear solved for a time. Then the problem appears again; another temporary solution. 'Botching' a job takes more effort in the long run because it will need doing and redoing regularly.

Option 3 is, of course, the cause-removing strategy. It takes more effort initially and sometimes courage to face up to reality, but it is permanent.

Permanent solutions need more effort in the short term,
but less in the long term, and they give peace of mind

I recently watched a television documentary which told the story of a 24-year-old American woman who weighed over 36 st. She was so overweight that doctors advised her that she was putting an unbearable strain on her heart. Her weight was killing her. In desperation she opted for surgery. A small pouch was constructed above her stomach which fooled the brain into thinking the stomach was full after only a few mouthfuls of food. She had to bear three years of painful treatment and she eventually lost over 24 st. Unfortunately that was not the happy ending.

She felt alone. She turned to drugs and alcohol to dull her emotional pain. It was then revealed that she had suffered sexual abuse as a child and had a very poor relationship with her mother. The documentary stated that modern medicine can treat only the symptoms and not the deep underlying causes. My experience supports this view. This case is an extreme example, but illustrates this point with poignancy.

UNDERSTANDING THE CONSCIOUS
AND THE SUBCONSCIOUS

I suggested earlier that you almost certainly do not know the full cause of your eating problem. By 'you' I am referring to the conscious you. Your subconscious may know exactly why food is causing difficulties.

Most of our memories and past emotions remain in our subconscious. It is like a giant filing system or a massive computer data bank. Our conscious minds usually have limited access to the wealth of stored information, which results in most people's memories being way less than 100 per cent.

The events in childhood have, to a large extent, moulded our personalities. There are genetic factors as well, but these are fixed at birth. All the rest has been learnt along the way.

Because few of us can consciously remember our early influences, it follows that most of us do not know why we are the way we are.

We do not know how our personalities have been moulded. For people with perfect personalities (I haven't met one yet) perhaps there is no need to look back – one could just enjoy living in the present. But for the rest of us, especially those with nagging difficulties in their life, it is important to understand why certain behaviour patterns came into existence.

If we return to the wallpaper example, it is impossible to find the cause of the damp if you stay inside the house. However, once you step outside, the wider perspective reveals vital new information – a slate is missing. This knowledge leads to a clear solution, although one, of course, still requiring effort.

This programme is designed to give you a wider perspective on yourself, by bringing certain subconscious memories to conscious awareness and giving you new ways of looking at eating problems.

As well as acting as a massive storage system, two other aspects of the subconscious are relevant here:

1 The subconscious protects

Emotions or events which are too painful for the conscious mind to cope with are locked away in the subconscious. These emotions and events are very important since they can *dictate behaviour* because the subconscious tries not to let similar pain happen again. To illustrate this, do you remember the first time that you burnt your fingers? Probably not. But your subconscious doesn't waste time in moving your hand off a very hot object. You don't even have to think about it. This is a wonderful protection mechanism.

However, the subconscious can also try to protect you from emotional pain which existed in childhood, but no longer exists. *This causes unwanted 'irrational' behaviour.* For example, suppose a child at primary school was ridiculed because of her different accent, emotional pain would have been experienced every time that child opened her mouth in the classroom. The subconscious would want to protect her from this pain. One strategy it could use would be to give the child such unpleasant anxiety feelings every time she was about to speak in front of other people that she would not even try. In fact, she would avoid such situations wherever possible. (This example, like most others I have included, is based on a real case.)

This protective mechanism could persist into adulthood, which would cause this person great difficulties. She might still feel anxious when speaking in groups, even though nobody ridiculed her accent any more.

The protective mechanisms of childhood can become
the restricting irrational behaviour of adulthood

I believe that we all have some of these restrictions. They can be removed – I have seen it happen time and time again. This programme will help you remove yours, particularly those that concern eating.

2 The subconscious needs commanding

If the subconscious was intelligent, it would realize when to stop certain strategies which have become redundant because of changed circumstances. The evidence suggests that the subconscious does not think in the logical way that the conscious mind does. The subconscious thinks by association. It works by making many neuro-mental associations. If you fall in love while dancing to a particular piece of music, that music will be associated with lovely feelings – often for the rest of your life.

Childhood associations can remain right through adult life, unless something powerful happens to change the habitual way of behaving. You will learn later in the programme how to powerfully command unwanted associations to cease.

EXERCISE

To demonstrate how stored memories can come up to the surface:

- Can you remember your first day at school?
- How clear is the memory?
- Are there any emotions attached to the memory?
- How about school dinners?
- What did you like?
- What did you detest?
- Are there any smells or tastes associated with school dinners?
- Do you remember the dinner ladies . . . ?

I would guess that you had many memories pop back into your mind when answering these questions. Did some of those memories have

18

emotions associated with them? What were those emotions? Were some painful and some pleasurable? Whatever they were, they are unique to you. Nobody else will have exactly the same mix of memories and emotions. The neuro-mental associations you have are unique. That is why different people need different solutions to problems which, on the surface, may appear the same.

Your subconscious is the power base of your mind. When it is programmed with positive forces, your full potential will be available for you to enjoy. I hope you recognize how important it has been to cover this material before we delve into eating behaviour itself. Let's do that now.

THE SEXIST NATURE OF FAT

Have you ever wondered why diets are mainly directed towards women and not men? And why were 95 per cent of my eating-problem clients women?

Think of the different pressures a woman has to face in this society compared with a man. The image of the ideal woman goes something like this (according to advertising agents):

- slim
- elegant
- innocent
- sensual
- vulnerable
- successful
- good housekeeper
- good mother
- good wife
- good cook
- responsible
- fun

The next time the adverts are on, try to add some more 'ideal characteristics'.

Looking through the above list you will find mutually exclusive characteristics. So the image is virtually impossible to attain, even if you wanted to attain it. It is bad enough to be pressured into conforming to any image, but when that image is self-contradictory, and therefore impossible to reach, the effects are feelings of failure and inadequacy.

Pressure starts at a young age

Women are generally taught to see themselves as men-catching objects. This starts at a young age and builds momentum as girls get older. Think of all the teenage magazines that start the preoccupation with page after page of boyfriend-getting advice. Fashions, make-up, anti-spot cream and diets then take on real importance. What happens for many young women is that they have lost control of their body even before their bodies have stopped growing. A friend of mine told me that when she was at school you had 'made it' if you could get into size 8 jeans. And if you couldn't . . . ?

Many teenage girls are not overweight – but they start believing that they are when they compare themselves with ultra-slim models (many of whom have anorexic tendencies). A recent survey showed that 40 per cent of teenage girls considered themselves overweight. Teenagers are particularly self-conscious and become fascinated and preoccupied with their bodies. If they start dieting at this stage when they are not actually overweight, it will be a real struggle. The deprivation will have started which often leads to overeating as a compensation, and the vicious circle begins.

Now it is time for you to start reflecting and remembering back to your youth. In the space below write down how you felt about your body during your teenage years.

NOTE: This is where the workbook starts. I cannot stress enough how vital it is to write things down and not just have a few fleeting thoughts. The amount of time you invest here and in each of the practical exercises will dramatically alter the effectiveness of the programme.

As a teenager, I felt my body was _____

_____

_____

_____

Who moved the goal posts?

The required image does not stay constant. Fashions change annually. The ideal body image seems to go in decades. In the 1950s there was the full, curvy Marilyn Monroe shape to copy. Then came the beanpole shape of Twiggy in the 1960s, to be followed by the permed hair and large breasts of Raquel Welch in the 1970s. Then came the tall and slim Princess Diana. Then in the 1990s back to the waif-like Kate Moss.

So what is the ideal woman? Of course, there is no ideal. The ideal is based on media hype, fashion and profit-driven motives.

Brainwashing

Over the last few decades, one consistent message has been broadcast:

To be beautiful is to be thin

This message is so powerful and pervasive that it amounts to brainwashing. I received a summer edition mail-order catalogue through the post recently which was 32 pages long. It managed to cram in 44 photographs of slim women in swimsuits. They were draped over barbecues, garden hoses, car vacuum cleaners; you name it, they were showing it off in a swimsuit. It is not surprising that many women – perhaps you – succumb to this pressure and struggle towards the ultra-thin image. Other women strongly reject these images – are you in this second category? Or perhaps you have a foot in both camps. Do you outwardly reject these images, but inside hanker to look like a model?

What about men?

Men have different pressures from women, and I think it will be interesting and valuable for you to appreciate the effects of these pressures.

The image-conscious 1980s created the ideal man, who should be:

- shrewd
- tough
- wealthy
- successful
- driving an expensive car
- wearing fashionable clothes
- handsome

- tall
- thin
- fit

Designer man arrived. The boom in male cosmetics and fitness clubs was a sign of the trend. In more recent years the ideal 'new' man has to be sensitive, supporting and a nappy-changer as well.

The price

Chasing imposed images takes its toll on men as well as women, and because the ideal body image is fit and lean, food and exercise become involved.

Eating disorder clinics which never saw a male patient ten years ago are now admitting a significant number of city professionals. Anorexic men are now not uncommon. Men in one way have it harder than women. They are supposed to be tough and have no weakness, so find it harder to admit to having an eating problem. They usually do so only when forced to through serious illness. So women are not the only casualties of the image makers.

Now let's return to women and consider motherhood.

Motherhood

As a wife and mother, a woman has a new ideal image to strive for.
The perfect wife and mother should:

- put her family's needs before her own;
- keep the house clean and tidy;
- provide popular meals at regular times;
- comfort and love her children;
- buy food and clothing within a budget;
- look after her husband by
  - satisfying him sexually;
  - being a social and business asset;
  - knowing where he put his newspaper;
  - supporting his ideas;
  - nursing him when he is ill.
- Still do all the above if she works.

Women often judge themselves to be failures if they do not achieve 100 per cent in all these areas, with the resulting stress of trying to achieve, followed by lowering of confidence when it becomes impossible.

BE YOURSELF

Perhaps your first step is to reclaim your mind from the brainwashing. This takes courage and maturity because we have to reject what society is telling us. Breaking away from what we 'should be' to who we are is a vital part of reclaiming your sense of personal power.

IS YOUR FAT TRYING TO SAY SOMETHING?

The idea is dynamite:

Your fat may be trying to help you

This might seem crazy, but I have found this to be so for many problem eaters, particularly compulsive eaters. It may not apply to you, but if it does it could be the key to the solution.

Case Study 1

Let's examine this idea in a case history. Meet Daisy Platen, an outwardly confident young woman who was pursuing a career in human resources. She happened to have blonde hair.

As a teenager Daisy was bombarded by the messages: get thin to be attractive and get a good job. She got a good job and wanted to be thin. However, her subconscious had made the association between looking attractive and being treated as a 'dumb blonde'.

Her subconscious made her eat so that she would get fat to neutralize her attractiveness. Her fat was trying to help her! It believed she could not be both career-minded and attractive. It is vital to realize that this was a subconscious process. Daisy consciously wanted to be thin. When subconscious and conscious are in conflict, an inner battle wages and disturbing behaviour – such as compulsive eating – can result.

When Daisy made a real effort to lose weight she successfully lost $1\frac{1}{2}$ st. She then began to notice that the behaviour of her male colleagues started to change. They began to be more interested in what she was doing in the evenings rather than her ideas about the new salary structure. In a way it was pleasing to her, but she wanted to be taken seriously in her work.

The solution for Daisy was to assert her right to be listened to, whether fat or thin

She learnt how to be firm with the men at work, so that they treated her primarily as a worker and only secondarily as a woman. When she did this her fat was made redundant, and she no longer felt a compulsion to eat when not hungry. She *could* have a satisfying career and be thin. This is a classic example of the psychological solution to an eating problem.

After the next case study, there is an exercise which should help you decide whether or not your fat is trying to be of service to you.

Case Study 2

This case study also sees fat in the context of sexuality.

Angela was 32 and married to Geoff; they had no children yet, although they both wanted to start a family soon.

Angela had suffered from bouts of compulsive eating for about three years, which started about a year after her marriage to Geoff. When she came to see me she was about 2 st above her weight on her wedding day. Her worst time for eating was in the evenings. She just couldn't stop herself going for the biscuit tin. When she didn't buy biscuits, it was bread and jam. One evening when the biscuits and bread had run out, she went to the local shop and bought a cake mix, and baked a jam sponge. This evening was one of the many evenings that Geoff was out working in a pub. When the cake had come out of the oven she had one piece, then another, and another, until it was half gone. She felt bloated, with a sense of self-disgust and despair about being out of control. She became worried about what Geoff would think if he came home and found a half-eaten cake. She often felt guilty about overeating. So she wrapped the remaining cake in a brown paper bag, and went outside and put the bag in a neighbour's dustbin. The next day she telephoned to make an appointment to see me.

Having heard her history, I asked her the following question: 'What might happen to you if you were slim?'

After a few positive responses such as 'I could wear prettier clothes', 'I'd feel happier about exposing my body in the swimming pool', and 'I'd feel much healthier', there came the following answer:

'Well, sometimes I think that if I was more attractive, I may get a lot more attention from some of my old boyfriends. I used to have no problem getting boyfriends, you know. But I have a good marriage, a nice house, I love Geoff and I want children. I don't want to risk losing these things by messing around with other men.'

I then asked her if there were aspects of her marriage that she would like to change. Angela immediately replied, 'I love Geoff, but I'm not sure he loves me.'

Further discussion revealed that, as well as having a job during the day, Geoff worked four evenings a week in a pub. He had started working like this about three years earlier in order to afford the monthly payments on a new car. Angela started off by going to the pub with Geoff, but soon got bored sitting at the bar, managing only brief words with him between customers.

Angela described how she was feeling in need of love and affection, and Geoff wasn't at home often enough to give them. She suspected Geoff thought more about the pub and the car than he did about her. So feelings of jealousy and rejection were there too. These emotions were making her vulnerable to having an affair. She could no longer trust her fidelity. *So her fat was ensuring that she stayed faithful* by discouraging approaches in the first place.

You may wonder why Angela did not just talk to Geoff about her feelings. Well, it was the terrible twins of low self-esteem and guilt. Her low self-esteem made her think, 'Oh well, I can't be that lovable if he prefers to go to work,' and the guilt worked something like this: 'I don't want to be one of those nagging wives – a man needs his freedom.'

By understanding the underlying causes of her eating problem, she realized how important it was to resolve the dissatisfaction with her husband. To help her do this, I gave her the material contained in Part 3 of this programme to read at home.

A week later, at the following session, she told me that she had followed the guidelines, summoned up the courage, and told her husband that she wanted him at home more often. She told me how surprised she was at his reply, 'Why didn't you tell me before? You said nothing, so I assumed you liked me out of your way.'

Geoff agreed to cut down his evening work and extend the payments on the car. They fell in love again and began talking much more to each other. Angela's fat was redundant now that her faithfulness was no longer in question.

She lost about 3 lb per week without even trying, simply because the compulsion to eat had gone, and then stabilized at her wedding-day weight.

Angela's problem was solved when she asserted her needs

More on assertiveness in Part 3.

Battle inside the mind

It may be difficult to grasp that your eating habits may be caused by a subconscious desire to be fat, but I hope you are beginning to see a possible connection.

When the conscious desire to be slim is in conflict with a subconscious strategy to be fat, there is an inevitable battle. The subconscious mind is very powerful, so it is a battle which the conscious mind rarely wins.

This struggle leads to the bizarre behaviour of many problem eaters. For example, in front of friends they may be the perfect dieter, but with guilt-ridden eating going on in secrecy. Friends may say, 'I don't know how you put weight on, you never eat.'

I don't intend to delve into the self-disgust, suffering and habits of problem eaters. I have never found that wallowing in misery helped clients at all. Hours and hours of talking about symptoms does not solve problems, it just creates depression. New perspectives solve problems.

One of the new perspectives presented here is that instead of seeing subconscious urges as the enemy, we try to understand them and *create co-operation* between subconscious and conscious.

The next exercise may help you come to such an understanding.

EXERCISE

Fat/thin fantasy
I suggest reading through the following fantasy twice so that you can close your eyes and remember the imaginary sequence.

Get as comfortable as you can ... Close your eyes ... and imagine yourself at a party ... You are getting fatter ... you are now quite large ... What does it feel like? ... Take a note of your surroundings ... How do you feel about them? ... What kind of party is it? ... What kinds of activities are going on? ... Notice whether you are sitting or standing, or moving about ... What are you wearing and how do you feel about your clothes? ... What are they expressing? ... Observe all the details in this situation ... How are you interacting with the other people at the party? ... Are you on your own or talking, dancing, eating with others? ... Do you feel like an active participant or do you feel excluded? ... Are you making the moves to have contact with others or are the other people at the party seeking you out? ... Now see what this 'fat' you is saying to the people at the party ... Does it have any specific messages? ... Does it help you out in any way to be fat in this situation? ... See if you can go beyond the feelings of revulsion you might have, to locate any benefits you see from being this size at the party ...

Now imagine all the fat peeling and melting away, and in the fantasy you are as thin as you might ever like to be ... You are at the same party ... What are you wearing now? ... What do these clothes convey about you? ... How do you feel in your body? ... Do you feel more or less included now? ... Are people approaching you or are you making the first moves? What is the quality of your contact with others? ... See if you can locate anything scary about being thin at the party ... See if you can get beyond how great it feels and notice any difficulties you might be having with being this thin ... Now go back and forth between the two images and particularly notice the differences ...

Now write down your feelings and any discoveries that you have made during this exercise:

_____

_____

_____

_____

_____

If any aspect of your fantasy became more comfortable when you were fat, you have found at least one underlying cause of your eating problems.

(I am grateful to Susie Orbach, author of *Fat is a Feminist Issue* (3rd edn, Arrow 1998), who used the above exercise in her eating therapy groups.)

Many of my clients initially had negative reactions when they got fatter, such as feeling like a lump of lard or self-loathing. Then, after the initial unpleasant reactions, many clients began to discover the positive things that being overweight was giving them, such as:

'I felt safe – I wasn't being eyed up.'

'I became more friendly and happy.'

'People were listening to me.'

'I was able to sit and relax – no pressure to perform.'

'I wasn't in competition with other women.'

'I was me.'

'I felt stronger and more substantial.'

If, during the fat/thin fantasy, you felt totally comfortable with the thin you, it shows that your fat is doing nothing for you in that particular fantasy setting. Before we assume that your fat is not doing anything for you, repeat the fantasy, but change the scene. Choose a situation which could be uncomfortable for you – perhaps visiting your parents, your in-laws, your workplace, or perhaps with your husband and children.

Run through the full fantasy, changing from fat to thin, in each situation.

These exercises are vital to your understanding
of your problem. The more you put into them,
the more you will get out

Only move on to the next section when you can definitely answer the question, 'Is your fat doing something for you?'

If the answer is 'yes', then write it down below:

My fat is trying to _____

_____

_____

If you have written an answer above, it will give you a clear indication of what changes you have to make in order to solve your weight/eating problem. Part 3 will show you how to make these changes that will enable you to take over what your fat is trying to do for you now. There may be other deep emotional causes. They often have their roots in the family.

From generation to generation

A recurring theme from client to client was their relationship with their mother. Let's explore the daughter/mother relationship.

Your mother provided you with a model for your behaviour as a woman. Your mother's behaviour was moulded on her mother, and all these behaviours were influenced by the expected role of women in society at the time. Most girls used to believe that their role was one of giving and supporting others, rather than developing their talents in a self-directive way. Often girls were not encouraged to study for exams, and this closes many doors into professional careers. This has changed in recent years, but if you are of a generation that was conditioned into the caring and supporting role, you may still associate yourself primarily with that role.

The mother's central role, nurturing and feeding her children, often becomes exaggerated because there seems to be little else in her life. A mother's reason for being is often solely for her children. Without her children, what does she have left? So there is a conflict: a need to see her children develop and become independent and a requirement still to be needed by her children.

This need to be needed can lead to a mother's being over-protective towards her children. This inevitably causes lowered self-confidence in her children. An over-protective mother often over-feeds her children in over-zealous nurturing. This introduces poor eating habits at an early age.

Mothers who resent their central role being taken away may use guilt as a strategy to keep their children dependent on them. (One of my clients told me that unless she visited her mother every day, her mother would sulk for days.)

If you are made to feel guilty, your self-esteem drops

From the daughter's point of view there is also possible conflict: a desire to become free and independent but a reluctance to do so because women still do not have equality in society. (One anorexic client expressed a fear that if she achieved too much in her life, it would be going one better than her mother whom she did not want to hurt.)

Other ways of being overweight which can be caused by the mother/daughter relationship are:

- a rebellion against the mother's wishes for a 'perfect' daughter: the fat is a powerful way of expressing the daughter's need to be independent from her mother;
- a way of saying to a mother, 'I can't cope on my own, you are still needed to be my mother.'
- a way of showing Mum how substantial her daughter is: 'I am big enough to look after myself.'

Explore the relationship you have, or had, with your mother, focusing on any areas of conflict, and try to discover if eating, being fat, and food have been influenced by these conflicts. Write down your thoughts:

_____

_____

_____

_____

_____

_____

_____

_____

Fat and fear of failure

For some women being fat is expressing their fear of failure. This fear may be conscious or subconscious. Do you ever hear yourself saying things like:

'I could get a job if it wasn't for being overweight.'
or:
'When I've lost weight, then I'll start getting fit.'
or:
'I would be in the mood for sex more often if I was thin.'

There are endless examples. Being overweight can be a convenient thing to blame for failing, or not even trying. If this blaming is caused by a fear of failing, then until the fear is removed, the fat excuse will be needed. The fat is doing something useful.

What do you commonly say that you will do when you are slimmer? Write down your answers.

_____

_____

_____

_____

_____

Now look back at your answers and circle those that have an element of fear or anxiety attached to them.

The answer to fear of failure is self-confidence and self-esteem. Have you noticed how confident people will try anything, and accept that they may fail (although their positive attitude means they rarely do)?

Part 3 should help if you fall into this category.

COMFORT EATING

We all need emotional nurturing: tender loving care (TLC).

If we don't receive enough TLC from people, we often seek it from food. After all, at the very earliest age a baby associates TLC with being fed. Food is associated again with emotions when children are given sweets for being 'good', or as a bribe to be 'good', or to take their mind off something painful. (I still remember being praised for my bravery and given a toffee by a nurse when I had to have stitches in a cut when I was four years old.)

Remember your own childhood. Write down below when and why treats (sweets, chocolate, cakes, biscuits, crisps, etc.) were given to you. Look for the emotional link:

31

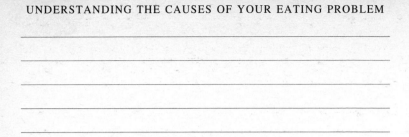

Eating to smother emotions

Food can be used to make up for a lack of pleasant emotions, and also to smother unpleasant emotions.

If you have emotions rising to the surface, such as anger, guilt or depression, eating can be a way to avoid experiencing these difficult emotions. The stronger and more difficult the emotions are, the more the mind may concentrate on food. A binge is the extreme strategy whereby eating blots everything else out.

Let's imagine you are feeling depressed about some aspect of your relationships and you turn to food. The food may provide some comfort and also take your mind off the depression. This strategy is, of course, only temporary and has unwanted side-effects (your weight). Moreover, *it is an avoidance of the real problem.*

The real problem lies inside you, and cannot be properly solved by temporary comforters and distracters.

If you do not know how to change yourself it is understandable for you to turn to any helper.

Do any of the following emotions play an ongoing part in your life, and how comfortable are you when thinking about them?

- guilt
- fear
- anger
- jealousy
- hurt
- depression
- despair
- insecurity
- rejection
- loneliness

Do you turn to food to smother these emotions? List the emotions you find most difficult to cope with. (Don't restrict yourself to the above list.)

_____

_____

_____

_____

_____

_____

In Part 3, you will learn how to take control of your emotions, which will make eating to smother them a thing of the past.

The meaning of food in childhood

You have already done the exercise at the beginning of this section, which asked you to think about food treats in childhood. But as well as food being associated with love and comfort, it can be associated with other powerful influences.

Do any of the following statements start bells ringing from your childhood:

'It doesn't matter if you are hungry or not, you are not leaving the table until you have finished your dinner.'
(This links the emotion of fear to listening to body messages.)

'Girls are made of sugar and spice and all things nice.'
(If you add 'you are what you eat' you get FOOD = SUGAR.)

'No pudding until you've finished the first course.'
(This encourages a negative attitude to savoury food because nobody likes being forced. It also encourages eating when not hungry, and reinforces sweet food as a reward.)

'Waste not, want not.'
(This encourages eating when not hungry, by using guilt to ensure nothing is left, hungry or not.)

Children brought up when rationing was in force, from large poor families or any home where food was in short supply, often still eat each meal as though it was their last, quickly and completely.

This is just a selection of a few childhood influences which may affect adult eating patterns. Obviously your own influences are unique. The next exercise will help you to clarify them.

> ## EXERCISE

Childhood eating memory trip

Read the following exercise through a couple of times, then close your eyes and go through the whole memory trip.

Go back somewhere between your fifth and tenth birthday ... Recall the house you were living in ... the kitchen ... your bedroom ... See the faces of the rest of your family as they were then ... Remember meals that brought the family together – maybe Sunday lunch ... Was the atmosphere tense or relaxed ... ? How are your mum and dad behaving towards you ... ? How are you behaving ... ? How are you eating the food ... ? Pay attention to other members of your family ... You may be receiving messages linked to food ... Stay with the memory and explore what is happening for as long as you need.

Write down below what you have learnt about the associations that were made with food from your childhood:

_____

_____

_____

_____

_____

_____

_____

_____

_____

As discussed earlier, the young subconscious mind accepts many things which are false. It cannot reason and be selective the way you can now. So it is time to go through the above list and decide which food neuro-mental associations are no longer valid. For example, if you were made to 'eat it all up – hungry or not', you may want to change that message to 'I will stop eating when I am satisfied' or 'Leaving food is better than eating too much.'

To make each new message sink in repeat it out loud with a firm voice at least ten times, and each time add 'The old message is now gone.' AFTER THE REPETITIONS, PICTURE, IN YOUR IMAGINATION, THE NEW WAY IN ACTION

List the new messages you want to give yourself:

_____

_____

_____

_____

EATING CHANGES
DURING AND AFTER PREGNANCY

During pregnancy

- '*Hooray, the fat won't show*' is a common reaction. If a woman has spent a long time struggling with her eating, pregnancy can be nine months of wonderful eating to make up for all the deprivation that has gone on before – with the fat not showing.
- '*Have some more, you are eating for two now.*' Other people can encourage a pregnant woman to eat when it is not necessary, unless she has the confidence to assert, 'No thanks, I'm trusting my body, and it tells me that I'm not hungry.'
- '*Who is having the baby – me or the hospital?*' If the health professionals seem to take over the pregnancy, feelings of resentment, lack of control and self-doubt could lead to comfort eating.
- '*Can I cope with motherhood?*' Even with caring support it is not surprising for feelings of inadequacy to emerge, especially during a first pregnancy. This could lead to comfort eating.

If this section is relevant to you, write down your eating and emotional experiences during pregnancy, trying to make sense of them:

_____

_____

_____

_____

_____

_____

_____

Mother and baby

Many women find that they do not return to their pre-pregnancy weight, and some even keep gaining. Let's discuss some of the possible explanations.

- *'I haven't been out for six months.'* Looking after a baby is a radical change of lifestyle. The opportunities for exercise may have been lost. New opportunities have to be created to fit around the needs of the baby (e.g. jumping on an exercise bike when the baby is sleeping).
- *'I'm suffering from post-natal depression.'* This could lead to comfort eating, which may simply pass when the depression lifts. But if the mother has started to diet, the vicious circle of eating>dieting>eating>dieting may keep going on even when the depression has gone.
- *'I'm not ready to start making love again.'* If a woman feels unable to verbalize this wish to her partner, perhaps because she feels it her duty to satisfy his sexual needs, her subconscious could make her overeat to get fat, trying to look less desirable.
- *'You only visit to see your grandchild.'* During the pregnancy, the expectant mother is the centre of attention, but if her parents, in-laws, friends and husband focus all their attention on the new baby, Mum could feel rejected or jealous. So to comfort eating.

These are only some possibilities. If this section is relevant to you, explore the emotion/food link that occurred after pregnancy:

_____

_____

_____

_____

SUMMARY OF THE UNDERLYING
EMOTIONAL AND PSYCHOLOGICAL
CAUSES OF EATING PROBLEMS

1 **Pressure to conform to society's ideal image**
   ('Very thin is beautiful' – obsessive dieting leading to compulsive eating.)
2 **Fat making subconscious statements**
   (I'm substantial, I'm not conforming, I'm not available, I still need you Mum, etc.)
3 **Comfort eating as a substitute for love**
   (I love chocolate and it is always available.)
4 **Comfort eating to smother unpleasant emotions**
   (Food rather than loneliness or anxiety.)
5 **Food-associated messages in childhood**
   (Waste not, want not. Eat up – or else . . .)
6 **Poor eating and lifestyle habits that have become ingrained**
   (It is easier to stay with old familiar patterns.)

CONCLUSIONS TO PART 2

Eating problems are caused by inappropriate neuro-mental associations. There are two types of NMA:

- _habitual NMA_: this is an NMA without an emotional link. For example, you have got in the habit of grabbing high fat or sugar snack foods, rather than eating a balanced meal. You see the crisp packet, then you are eating the crisps almost before you know it. The issue here is to increase the motivation and determination to break the old habit.
- _emotional NMA_: this is an NMA with strong emotion attached to it. The food or the fat is trying to satisfy your emotional needs. If

you try to do without the food or the fat, painful feelings emerge. You feel bad when you eat, you feel bad when you don't. The issue here is to satisfy your emotional needs without the need for food. Food then becomes the way you nourish your body and will give you pleasure as you taste nutritious foods.

Your conclusions

What are your own conclusions? What have you learned about you and your relationship with food and eating? Have you uncovered the underlying cause of your eating problem? Please write your conclusions here:

_____

_____

_____

_____

_____

_____

_____

PART 3

The Psychological and Practical Solutions

Introduction

The work you have done in Part 2 should have given you a clear insight into the cause of your eating problem. This knowledge itself may make you feel better. Knowledge takes you out of the helpless zone and into the realm of solutions. But just being in this realm does not guarantee success. You have to decide what you have to do and then *take action*.

Some people, having discovered the causes of the problem, are apprehensive about making changes that will fundamentally change their lives. That is understandable because most people associate change with the fear of going into the unknown. The fear of failure may loom large as well. That is why Part 3 concentrates on building self-esteem first of all, which will then give you the confidence to make the changes necessary. Once you have more self-esteem and confidence you will be able to start changing the way you get your emotional needs satisfied. Then we shall work through the section on changing habits. Finally, there is the ten-week action plan which will help you focus on achieving your goals.

If you decide that you want to change your life, you will need to expend energy. This effort will be challenging and rewarding if you are self-motivated. Self-motivation needs desire. Cultivate your motivation to change your life for the better by thinking about your desire to change many times a day. Go to sleep thinking, 'I want to change, I will change . . .'

INCREASING YOUR SELF-ESTEEM

Self-concept: Who do you think you are?

Your self-concept is made up of your beliefs, attitudes and self-esteem. For example, if you believe 'Women do not make good car mechanics', this belief will become part of your self-concept, the way you see yourself. So you think, 'I would not make a good car mechanic because I am a woman.' With this thought in your mind, how do you think you would approach a car which did not start? Not with a great deal of confidence. So:

Your beliefs become your reality

An experiment was carried out in a school in the USA. The headteacher invited three teachers into her office at the beginning of the school year. She told the teachers that they were each going to have a class of significantly higher IQ pupils that year. They were delighted, looking forward to a stimulating and rewarding group of pupils. In reality these teachers were going to teach pupils of just average IQ.

At the end of the year, the exam grades of these three classes were significantly above the rest of that year's classes, and the individual IQ scores had also significantly increased.

In the headteacher's office after the results had been announced, the three teachers were reflecting on how good it had been to teach such intelligent students. Then the headteacher told them that they were singing the praises of average IQ students and that they had been deceived as part of an experiment.

The teachers realized that their beliefs changed their expectations, which in turn changed their behaviour. They were more enthusiastic, more patient, more encouraging, etc. This behaviour brought out the best in their students, who in fact became what the teachers believed them to be. *Belief became reality.*

People used to believe the world was flat. Sailors believed they would sail off the edge of the earth. In their reality the earth was flat. They experienced real fear when they thought they were sailing close to the edge.

This leads to the conclusion:

Change your beliefs, change your reality

How was your self-concept formed?

A young baby is:

1 fearless – they try anything and everything;
2 uninhibited – they express themselves spontaneously.

As a baby grows, learning takes place by:

1 imitation – they copy their parents;
2 seeking pleasure – they do what feels good;
3 avoiding pain – they don't do what hurts.

As babies experiment, they want to touch everything within reach. This uninhibited curiosity is, for most babies, met with a good deal of 'Stop! No. You can't! Dirty!' etc. The repeated restraining of a baby's natural curiosity may lead to 'I can't' feelings. This is coupled with fear of disapproval and apprehension.

Babies are punished for doing things which are natural

I am not suggesting that babies ought to be left to injure themselves. They may be stopped, but should not be punished for behaving naturally. The best way to stop them is to divert them to something more interesting. This takes thought, time and patience. Even the best parents are sometimes going to be tired and lose patience. So all of us, as babies, have had our natural and uninhibited behaviour restricted to some extent, our self-concept tinged with 'I can't.'

Parental rejection

Self-concept is certainly going to be the casualty when a child is rejected in some way by a parent.

Rejection can come in many forms. Here are several possibilities:

- favouritism shown to brothers or sisters;
- lack of interest or time given to the child;
- lack of love and affection;
- other activities coming before the child;
- violence inflicted by a parent to the child.

Sometimes there is no actual rejection, but a perceived rejection. In fact it doesn't matter whether there is real rejection or not: if rejection is perceived, then self-concept will suffer. For example, a friend of mine was sent to boarding school and felt somewhat rejected. It wasn't until 20 years later, when chatting to his parents, that he discovered the real reason. He was dyslexic, which makes reading and writing difficult, and his parents sent him to a private boarding school which encouraged dyslexics. At the time state

41

schools treated dyslexics as though they were low in intelligence, which is not true.

So he now realizes that, rather than rejecting him, his parents sacrificed a great deal to give him a good start in life. As a child he did not understand the actions of his parents and misinterpreted them, with the resultant doubt over his self-worth. His new perspective on those past events is of great significance to him as it has changed his image of himself and his parents.

Of course, sometimes rejection is real, with no hope of later discovering that it had all been a dreadful misinterpretation. When rejection is perceived, it often leads to a fear of rejection in later life.

If you suffered rejection, it is vital to realize that just because you have been rejected in the past, it does not follow that you are an unworthy, unlovable person. When we are very young, we see our parents as infallible gods. They provide everything. Therefore we reason in a childlike way that, if they reject us, we are the ones who are to blame. They cannot be bad, so it must be us. Of course, as adults, we know that our parents are not perfect, and perhaps it is now time to stop blaming ourselves and to start accepting ourselves and our parents as we and they actually are.

Conditional pleasure

In search of good feelings, a young child learns to adapt its behaviour. Unfortunately, most parents use the following strategies:

'Mummy will give you a cuddle when you've been on the potty.'
'If you do that, Daddy will get angry.'

These seemingly harmless statements contain an implied message:

'You are not loved and safe unless you do what pleases Mummy and Daddy.'

If these messages are linked with a lack of love and little encouragement to explore and develop one's own identity, many children grow up believing they have to please Mummy, Daddy, brothers, sisters . . . and later, teachers, spouses and bosses. *This is caused by fear of rejection and leads to people being preoccupied by the wants of others.*

This restricted way of living is based on the belief: 'I am not loved and safe unless I do what X, Y or Z wants.'

If you are living your life by this belief, your life
will be only about 25 per cent of what it could be

It is vital to understand that *you can change your beliefs*. Just think how many of your beliefs have changed since you were 12 years old.

Traumatic incidents and self-esteem

People who were sexually abused as children or adults often have very low self-esteem. They often feel very guilty, soiled and unlovable. Professional one-to-one care may help them clear away this negative self-image.

Self-esteem

Self-esteem (SE) is the measure of how much you value and like yourself. SE can change with context. For example, you may have high SE at home and low SE at work.

Your SE is something inside you; it can't be seen. But it strongly influences your behaviour, which is like a beacon sending messages to everybody you meet. You can tell from a person's voice, their walk, their facial expressions whether they are happy or sad, confident or nervous.

Fill in the table on page 44.

Then ask yourself: Which list is the longer? Which was the easier to compile? Most people with eating problems have more in the low self-esteem column. By the end of this programme most people have a longer list in the high self-esteem column.

What I like about myself	What I dislike about myself
High self-esteem	**Low self-esteem**

Affirmations

Affirmations can help us understand and change our beliefs and boost our self-esteem. An affirmation is a strongly asserted positive statement that you would like to be a fact. Say out loud the following affirmations now:

> 'I can be loved and safe for being myself.'
> 'I can achieve anything I set my mind to.'

When you make these affirmations, what is the tone of your voice? If your voice is quiet and unsure, it shows that at the moment you don't really believe them to be true. The power of affirmations comes from the principle:

> *If you say anything long enough, you will start to believe it*

After all, this is how the false, negative messages were drummed into you in the first place.

> *Repeat the statements loudly and confidently*

Become aware of the power of voice tone and emphasis. Go back and repeat the statements rather quietly and feebly, then say them louder with enthusiasm and force. Now, what is closer to your normal voice, the firm or the feeble? Become aware of how important your voice tone is and practise speaking with a firm, confident voice.

> 'I can be loved and safe for being myself.'
> 'I can achieve anything I set my mind to.'

Self-image

Self-image describes how you see yourself. It includes how you see your body and your character.

Self-esteem is based on how much you like and value what you see. Therefore,

> *If you improve your self-image your self-esteem*
> *will automatically rise*

Self-image is essentially about how we label ourselves.

Labels are powerful things. Once labelled, anything can be put in its pigeon-hole.

> *You must resist the labels that other people try to impose on you. The first step is not to label yourself*

So, for example, if somebody asks you what you do, give them more than a label. If they show interest in you, explain what responsibilities and skills you have.

If you normally describe yourself as a 'housewife' you could say:

'I've been responsible for the physical and mental well-being of two children during their most formative years.'
'Now they are older, I give them advice about jobs and relationships. Even their friends ask me for advice.'
'I manage the household budget, make sure the bills are paid and we have enough saved for major items – and I do it all without a computer!'

(I don't really expect you to say all this, but keep this sort of positive self-image in your mind.)

After all, a housewife is a manager. The words used in business may sound impressive (time management, planning, delegation, decision-making, team motivation, etc.) but the so-called 'housewife' is doing these things all the time. She simply doesn't have the status symbols to go with them.

Just think of the impact you would have at a job interview if, instead of saying, 'I've been at home for the last seven years bringing up the children,' you gave an account of your skills and achievements during those seven years. One of my clients gained promotion and a pay rise three weeks after starting the programme, because her boss noticed the rise in her confidence in herself and her ability to deal with people. She also lost weight without a struggle.

Fill in the next page with your skills, responsibilities and achievements, throughout your whole life. Many people belittle their achievements, but just remember that what you now take for granted and find easy, at one time had to be learnt, be it cooking, word processing, driving, etc.

Modesty is a virtue, but self-deprecation is not. Blow your own trumpet for a while:

Self-appreciation sheet

From your whole life write down examples of:

YOUR SKILLS

_____

_____

_____

_____

_____

_____

_____

_____

YOUR RESPONSIBILITIES

_____

_____

_____

_____

_____

_____

_____

_____

YOUR ACHIEVEMENTS

_____

_____

_____

_____

_____

_____

_____

ASSERTIVENESS

Introduction

In Part 2, it was a recurring theme that most problem eaters need to assert themselves more. Do you remember the woman Daisy Platen, who was subconsciously using her fat to stop men making advances and to get them to take her seriously? When Daisy learnt to do that by using her mouth to say the necessary words, rather than using it to overeat, her problem was solved.

In this section you will discover that being assertive encourages positive emotions to start pouring into your life, and also stops the painful emotions from starting in the first place.

Learning to be assertive is another tremendous boost to self-esteem and self-confidence in almost every aspect of life.

The word 'assertiveness' is used to describe a certain kind of behaviour. It is a behaviour which helps us communicate clearly and confidently our needs, wants and feelings to other people, while at the same time respecting others' needs, wants and feelings.

So assertiveness focuses on your behaviour, which is an outside sign of self-esteem.

The three behaviours

It will help if we look at three types of behaviour: passive, assertive and aggressive. To recognize them, here are a few *non-verbal* signals that are shown in the three behaviours.

Passive

| Shuffling feet | Whining voice | Downcast eyes |

Assertive

| Upright, relaxed posture | Calm, controlled voice | Good eye contact |

Aggressive

| Pointing finger | Shouting | Staring eye contact |

The above descriptions are very brief, but you can probably recognize people you know who are habitually in each category.

Here are some words and phrases which go with the previous non-verbal signals of the three behaviours:

Passive

Sorry... Would you mind very much if... It's only me...
You decide... Well, I suppose I could... I couldn't do that...

Assertive

I feel like... What do you think... Let's talk...
I would like... I appreciate... No, I don't want to...

Aggressive

You stupid... If you don't... You must...
Just try it... You've done it again... Get lost...

Which behaviour best describes you?

Most of my weight-loss clients recognized that much of the time they exhibited passive behaviour, so we're going to concentrate on understanding passive behaviour before moving on to how to be assertive.

Passive behaviour

The causes

Some of the causes, based on low self-esteem, have already been covered, so I'll just briefly summarize them:

1 The 'I can't' and the spontaneity of babyhood restricted in early life.

2 Being conditioned by the meek and passive image and actual behaviour of women.
3 Learning that to conform is to be accepted.
4 The fear of trying anything new.
5 The fear of rejection.
6 The need for approval.

The prime importance of early conditioning, especially by one's parents, merits the next exercise:

EXERCISE

Here are some questions for you to answer. I have used Mother and Father because that is the most common. If you were brought up by your aunt and uncle, or whoever else, just change the heading. Answer either A (always), S (sometimes), or N (never).

	Mother	Father
Were you able to trust your parents?		
Did your parents give you encouragement and praise?		
Were you able to express your feelings openly?		
Did your parents make it clear that they loved you for who you were, and not for what you achieved?		
Did your parents demonstrate that they trusted you to make your own decisions as you grew up?		

You are indeed lucky if you can answer 'always' in all 10 boxes.

Not many people can. If you had a significant number of 'sometimes' and 'never' perhaps you can now understand your behaviour better. Each of us learned strategies to cope with the circumstances we were born into.

Although parents are the strongest influence for most people, brothers, sisters, teachers, the church, school, television all have a go at influencing us. Some influences help us to be free-thinking, confident people, while others restrict us and make us passive, or – with all that bottled-up anger – maybe aggressive.

Now you can include these influences in a little story – the story of the influences you received as a child. Write the story in the third person (i.e. There was a little girl and she had two brothers . . .). Writing in the third person, rather than saying 'I . . .', helps to separate the new you from the old conditioned you.

_____

_____

_____

_____

_____

_____

_____

_____

_____

_____

_____

_____

Domineering personalities

In your story, is there any figure who is a domineering personality (DP)? Is there a person you were frightened of or intimidated by, a person who you would never contradict, or could never win an argument with?

A DP may be strict and have a set of rigid rules which you break at the risk of heavy punishment or disapproval. Other DPs use the strategy of guilt to make people do what they want. Is there a DP in your life now? If so, do they make you feel inferior?

A DP may love their child very much and they may believe they are acting in the child's best interest. But the child often doesn't see it this way!

When faced with a difficult situation, the two instinctive responses are fight or flight. So the two 'knee-jerk' reactions to a DP are either to get aggressive and challenge them or to get out of their way to avoid conflict. It is more socially acceptable for a woman to adopt the latter strategy, which is being passive. Do you try to avoid conflict whenever possible?

*As thinking human beings we can rise above the
two instinctive reactions and learn to discuss, argue
and negotiate. This is being assertive*

Because assertiveness is not the natural response for most people, it has to be understood and practised, like any new skill. It is a bit like learning a new language.

Before you learn more about assertiveness, it is vital for you to agree that passive behaviour is not good for you.

Over-protective personalities (OP)

In contrast to domineering people are over-protective personalities. You can recognize OPs by the way they mollycoddle everyone – especially their children. They are always worrying whether their children will be hurt, emotionally or physically. If their child is home ten minutes late, they will be in a state of panic, on the point of ringing the police.

They like doing everything for their children, and they find it difficult to let their children grow up and become independent. Was there an OP in your story?

Parental over-protection can have profound effects on children.

1 They may believe they are not capable because they are not allowed to try anything demanding in case they fail or hurt themselves.
2 Everything they do is surrounded by a worrying parent, creating anxiety for the child.
3 They are so protected from life's knocks that they fear them all the more, often becoming conflict-avoiding adults.

The result is a child growing up with low self-esteem.

Passive behaviour case study

One of the strongest reasons why people behave passively is that they do not want to hurt other people. Let's consider an example.

Sue is a rather passive 25-year-old. Sue's best friend, Jane, was getting married and had been to dressmaking classes because she wanted to make her own wedding dress. Jane had finished the dress after weeks of work and was bubbling over with excitement and pride when she called round to show Sue the dress.

When Sue saw Jane wearing the dress she immediately noticed a rear seam that was not straight. But when Jane asked her verdict, Sue said, 'It looks great and you look wonderful.'

Sue did not want to hurt Jane's feelings.

Three hours before the wedding, Jane's mother arrived from the other end of the country, and of course wanted to see the dress on her daughter. Her mother asked, 'Has anyone seen the dress from the back . . . ?'

Jane was really angry. 'Why didn't Sue mention it? She must have seen it. I would have had time to correct it.'

When Jane expressed her anger to Sue, Sue could not stop apologizing and felt mortally guilty. In this example Sue didn't want to hurt Jane's feelings and so she was not honest with her. But in the end she ended up causing more hurt, both for Jane and herself. Do you think that Jane would ask for Sue's opinion again? What do you think happened to Sue's self-esteem?

Passive behaviour case study

A different example of being passive is made clear in the story of Judy's sexual relationship with her husband Peter.

Peter had found that all his previous girlfriends had enjoyed their ear lobes being nibbled. So when he met Judy two years ago, he started nibbling her ear. In fact, Judy did not like it at all – but she said nothing. Judy was scared of saying anything negative to Peter. It might hurt him . . . might he then reject her?

Because she had not said anything straight away, it became more and more difficult for her to mention it. In fact, she usually faked enjoyment. This had gone on for two years, and had made Judy sometimes avoid any affectionate cuddling.

One day, something quite trivial sparked off a row and

somewhere in the shouting match Judy screamed, 'And another thing, you don't even know what turns me on! I can't stand you chewing my ears!'

Peter was dumbfounded and there was a long silence before he found something to say. 'Why on earth didn't you tell me? I thought you enjoyed it.'

When they started talking about it, Peter was very understanding and was quite happy to nibble something else. Judy actually told him what she did like. Being passive on this one issue had caused two years of dissatisfaction.

Do you tell your partner what you like or how you want to be treated?

Being passive is not telling others what you like or want. One has to hope everyone is telepathic!

Fear

A common theme running through passive behaviour is fear: fear about what others may think, fear of hurting others, fear of looking or sounding silly, fear of conflict or fear of rejection.

Can you now understand that these fears were due to wrong early learning and low self-esteem? *You can eliminate these fears when you accept that they are false.*

It is time for the following affirmation:

> *'I can be loved and safe when being myself'*

Say it out loud. Proclaim it to yourself and to the world.

Guilt

Guilt is one of the most powerful forces that exists in many people's lives. It is especially common in passive people. But what exactly is guilt? Guilt is a self-punishment for believing that you have done something wrong. When you are on a diet and then eat something not allowed, you may feel guilty because you have done something 'wrong'. You broke the rule of your diet.

So the key to understanding guilt is to realize by what set of rules you live your life. For example, many mothers live by the rule: 'I should always put my needs behind the needs of my family.'

So, if they ever think about doing or buying something for themselves, they are threatening to break their rule and would feel guilty.

I hope you understand that these sorts of rules are all tied in with self-esteem. When self-esteem improves and you start standing up for your rights, your rules change, and so it is less often that you will feel that you have done something wrong. You will also start living by *the rules that you choose* rather than living by rules imposed from outside. There will be less need to punish yourself and that means less guilt.

Past guilt

Your rules contain your moral and ethical codes, which define your boundaries between good and bad behaviour. Many of my clients had a history of feeling guilty which stretched back a long way. Sometimes there was a particular event in the past that had so seriously broken an important rule that it was still causing guilt feelings.

Some of the events causing long-standing guilt that were told to me:

- having an abortion;
- not being present at the death of a parent;
- driving a car and knocking down a pedestrian;
- having a horse 'put down' by a vet;
- having an incestuous relationship;
- losing faith in God.

If you still feel guilty about something that happened a long time ago, please consider the next questions carefully. Have you punished yourself for long enough? Even armed gangsters are set free after serving a sentence. Does your self-imposed punishment really fit the 'crime'? Could you not forgive yourself, as you would forgive others?

If you would like to let go of long-standing guilt, do so now by acknowledging that you have learned from your mistakes and now forgive yourself:

I forgive myself for _____

I forgive myself for _____

Anger

Many passive people hardly ever express anger. They are frightened of doing so and try to avoid it.

In an ideal world, there would be no need to get angry. But anger does provide a useful service in certain circumstances. Anger lets people know that they are seriously infringing your rights or boundaries. It should be the reaction of last resort, after other assertive behaviour has been ignored, but it then becomes justified.

Some people will try to put you down and only stop when you get angry. Then they realize that they have gone too far.

Assertive people who get angry with a person are not rejecting that person, they are just letting them know that what they are doing, at that particular time, is very annoying. Assertive people can show anger to a person and still love them. Assertive people who show justified anger quickly forgive and forget.

In contrast, aggressive behaviour threatens a person, whereas angry behaviour shows that person how you feel.

Anger is best expressed at the time when you feel it rising. If it is bottled up, it can turn bitter and come out as aggression, biting sarcasm or malicious gossip, or the bitterness can turn inwards, with stress eating away at physical and mental health.

The first step is actually to express anger. It is better for you and it is also better for those around you, because anger is preferable to the effects of suppressed anger. When you accept that anger hurts others much less than bottled-up bitterness, the fear of expressing anger will disappear.

EXERCISE

Anger exercise
If the idea of expressing anger to another person is very difficult for you, start by letting your anger out when you are on your own. Get a pillow or cushion and shout at it, punch it, pour out all your suppressed anger. Release the pressure. Write a list of people, situations or events that have made you angry in the past and then a similar list of things which cause you anger now (and have the pillow ready):

The following made me angry in the past:

_____

_____

_____

The following makes me angry now:

_____

_____

_____

_____

_____

A lot of anger is anger at yourself. Passive behaviour often causes anger because you say to yourself things like, 'Why didn't I say a, b or c? Why didn't I do x, y or z?' So by being less passive, less anger and frustration will be directed towards yourself.

Summary of passive behaviour

How being passive can affect you

In the short term (the pay-offs):

- You feel a reduction of anxiety as you have avoided a possible conflict.
- You experience an escape from guilt feelings which you would have had if you had said 'no' to a request.
- You can always feel sorry for yourself: 'It's always me who gets landed with all the work.'
- You can feel proud, 'I take on so much, I hold the place together.'
- Others praise you for always putting yourself out for others.

But, in the long term, you experience:

- A growing loss of self-esteem.
- An increase in suppressed anger/frustration/hurt/self-pity.
- Internal tensions/stress and anxiety.
- Avoidance of difficult situations and decisions.
- Psychosomatic problems, e.g. headaches and backaches.

How being passive can affect others

The huge irony of passive behaviour is that when you try too hard to please others, you will rarely be appreciated and respected. If you do not respect yourself, you will rarely find others respecting you. Here are some of the effects of passive behaviour on others:

- Initially, others feel sorry for you.
- They feel guilty or indifferent (about taking advantage of you).
- They feel irritated (e.g. 'for goodness sake, *say* what you want').
- They find you boring (e.g. 'Do you always have to agree with me?').
- They cease to respect you.
- They restrict contact with you.

You should now be clear on the causes and difficulties of passive behaviour. If you think that some of your emotional eating is caused by long-term passive behaviour, you should now feel very motivated to do something about it.

How to be assertive

To be assertive we must:

- Decide what we want.
- Decide if it is fair.
- Ask clearly for it.
- Be unafraid of taking risks.
- Be calm and relaxed.
- Express our feelings openly.
- Give and take compliments easily.
- Give and take fair criticism.

And we should not:

- Bottle up our feelings.
- Beat about the bush.

In the context of eating problems, being assertive is about regaining the power that has been given to eating or to the fat

Rights

An assertive person realizes she has certain basic human rights. Each person has their own set of rights, depending on their choice, religion, culture and beliefs. The list below contains some of the most widely accepted ones:

1 To have opinions and feelings and to express them appropriately.
2 To ask for what we want (knowing that our request may be turned down).
3 To choose whether or not to get involved with the problems of another person.
4 To be treated as an equal, whatever our age, race, sex, class, religion, etc.
5 To say 'no' to requests that we don't want to comply with, without feeling guilty.
6 To make mistakes.
7 To say we don't understand, and ask for more information.
8 To change our minds.
9 To stand up for these rights and to make sure other people respect them.

With rights come responsibilities: *the assertive person respects the rights of others.* The passive person respects the rights of others, but does not stand up for her own. The aggressive person stands up for her own, but does not respect the rights of others.

Assertiveness is all about honest communication and compromise where both parties feel satisfied with the outcome

Behaviour breeds behaviour

A client, Margaret, would always stop whatever she was doing when her husband wanted a cup of tea. He hardly ever made tea; he said she made it much better than he did. Other people had told Margaret for years that 'her good nature' was being taken advantage of. When she was introduced to assertiveness, she recognized that what other people saw as her good nature was sometimes just a smiling façade, under which she did resent being taken for granted. Food sometimes smothered these emotions. She resolved to make some changes.

When she was genuinely busy she began saying to her husband, 'I'm in the middle of something now, can you put the kettle on?'

Initially her husband's reaction was sulky and he said that he couldn't be bothered – he didn't want a cup of tea that much anyway. At this point, Margaret began to feel guilty and nearly jumped up to make the tea. But she remembered our previous discussion, when I had explained that her husband might resist the changes. His sulking was an attempt to make her feel guilty, so that she would return to her usual passive behaviour.

If other people are on to a good thing (i.e. you are doing more than your fair share) then they will probably resist the change

If a person is generally unselfish, they will not resist your change much. In fact, they may feel guilty about taking advantage of you. However, if you have domineering personalities to deal with, they may resist your assertive behaviour quite strongly.

Sooner or later your new behaviour will make them change their behaviour and you will have earned their respect

You need determination and rising self-esteem to succeed in being assertive. The ten-week action plan will make it possible for you to succeed.

To finish the story about Margaret, she trusted my advice and didn't weaken. After two days of rather sulky behaviour from her husband, he actually asked her if she would like tea!

Perhaps more importantly, it started a discussion about him taking her for granted which led to real communication between them. Margaret's overeating had been caused by suppressed anger about being taken for granted.

Because passive people avoid conflict, they keep their displeasures to themselves, and these just build and build. This can result in an occasional explosion, which scares them, makes them feel guilty and leads them to over-apologize. This deepens fear of releasing emotions, so the vicious circle is completed. Alternatively, the suppressed emotions are kept so well locked in that passive people live their lives with a festering emotional sore eating away from the inside. This often causes physical illness. Food is frequently used to try to smother these painful emotions, or to produce fat that can be hidden behind.

The conflict that passive people try so hard to avoid is normally just in their imagination. This is because they usually only see two courses of action: to be either passive or aggressive. The aggressive action frightens them or seems completely alien to them, so the only option left is the passive one. Their reality has been created by the belief that one has to either shut up or shout out.

When this belief is changed by acting assertively, the imagined conflict often ceases to be there.

Why being assertive is good for your children

Let's return to Margaret. She also found that her assertiveness made her children respect her and listen to her. They used to wrap her around their little fingers. If she was cross with them, one little tear from her daughter would make her feel terribly guilty. She would apologize and give them a treat. (Just think what lessons her children were learning about manipulating.)

She realized that her guilt was rewarding their manipulative sulky behaviour. Every week they spent their pocket money on sweets on the first day, but they knew that they could get more out of Mum any time if they made her feel guilty by sulking or crying or getting angry. Margaret understood that giving in to this manipulative behaviour was creating two unpleasant children and lowering her self-esteem. So she decided to say 'no' once or twice. The children were very surprised and tried every trick in the book to make her feel guilty. Initially, she did feel guilty inside, but she knew that she mustn't show it. It was hard, but she realized why it was so important to ride the storm.

Now Margaret loves and cares for them just as much, but doesn't mollycoddle them. She has realized that by over-protecting them she was going to give them a very one-sided view of life. Mum would keep all the pain away from them and not let them learn from their own mistakes. Once out in the real world, her children would have got a shock when they realized that you can't always get what you want.

A simple description of assertiveness is: 'Firm but fair'

That is hardly a new idea. You can love people and still say 'no' to them.

The conclusion of Margaret's story

Margaret is now a happier, more confident person. Her husband, although not very good at talking about his emotions, has made it clear that he does love her and has started appreciating her more and pulling his weight around the house, though it took some weeks for this to happen.

Her children now usually do things when she asks the first time. They have stopped being sulky, because it does not work any more.

After a few days, the children had accepted that Mum had changed – so *they* changed. The whole family is now much closer because they actually communicate with each other.

Margaret lost 2–3 lb per week and stabilized at a weight she was comfortable with. There was no struggle, no dieting, she simply stopped eating the extra food which had helped smother her anger and frustration.

How do I know when I am not being assertive?

There is a very simple rule:

> *When we are assertive, our self-esteem rises*
> *When we are not assertive our self-esteem falls*

This means that although one of our rights is to express our opinions and feelings, it does not mean we have to. If, for diplomatic reasons, we keep our opinions to ourselves, that's fine. There is no loss of self-esteem if we keep our mouths shut for good reason. (In fact, the self-esteem would go down if we insensitively blurted out an opinion.) But when we keep quiet out of fear of being laughed at or rejected, then self-esteem suffers.

Being unassertive is walking away from a situation, saying to yourself, 'I wish I had said that . . .'

Tips on being assertive

• Have your body language in step with your words.

When you say, 'That's very kind of you, but I don't want to come in for coffee,' have a firm voice, upright posture and look the person in the eye.

• Be prepared not to get what you want.

Being assertive means that you ask for what you want. You may get all of what you want, some of it, or nothing at all.

When you ask, you are certainly more likely to receive than if you never ask. And even if you receive nothing, you feel you have at least tried, so your self-esteem does not suffer.

- Assertiveness is about saying 'yes' as well as 'no'.

We have concentrated on saying 'no' without feeling guilty. But this is not to imply that you stop saying 'yes'. It's lovely saying 'yes' when you genuinely want to. It's great to put yourself out for others, as long as you don't harbour resentment.

Coping with criticism

Most passive people crumple when faced with criticism. This is because it is a direct threat to their already low self-esteem. When you act assertively you boost your self-esteem and this changes your reaction to criticism in two ways:

1 To unfair criticism you stand your ground and put your opinion forward with firmness and confidence.
2 To justified criticism you accept it and actually appreciate the fact that you have been given a chance to improve what you are doing.

An assertive person admits when they are genuinely wrong

EXERCISE

Assertiveness profile

As mentioned earlier, the more assertive you are, the more comfortable you will feel in a given situation. So rate yourself from 0 to 10 (0 being very uncomfortable, 10 being totally comfortable) in the different situations below.

Activity	Comfort Rating	What are the effects of your level of comfort on you and your life?
Receiving compliments		
Expressing liking and love to another adult		
Making requests (e.g. asking for favours, help, etc.)		
Affectionate touching of another adult		
Initiating conversations with strangers		
Standing up for your rights (e.g. in a shop, with a neighbour, etc.)		
Refusing requests from family, work or friends		
Expressing personal opinions, including disagreeing		
Expressing anger		

Take plenty of time scoring your assertiveness profile, because it may provide the basis of some important changes you need to make. Perhaps it will be the first time you have ever looked at such a range of personal interactions.

As you fill in the profile, recognize that feeling comfortable is linked to feeling in control of the situation.

Many scores under 5 show that there are many areas of your life which create difficulties. Perhaps you avoid them. Practising assertiveness will help you increase these scores and help you to feel more in control of your life.

EXERCISE

Case study exercises

The following case studies give you an opportunity to understand what being assertive means in different situations. After each case study write down how you would have handled the situation in the past and how you will handle the situation now, with your knowledge of assertive behaviour. Write down exactly what you would say and do.

Situation 1

You are unexpectedly delayed on a train and you will be home later than expected. Your family will be worried about you. You do not have a mobile phone with you, but the person sitting opposite does. What do you do?

As your old self: _____

_____

_____

_____

As your new assertive self: _____

_____

_____

_____

Situation 2

A rather domineering friend has called round to see you. You wanted to get to the shops before they close, and you are not very interested in what your friend is saying. She does not seem to be going, and unless you end the conversation now, the shops will have closed. What do you say and do?

As your old self: _____

_____

_____

_____

As your new assertive self: _____

_____

_____

_____

Situation 3

You are in bed with your husband/boyfriend. He starts touching you in ways that usually mean he wants to make love. However, you don't want to. You don't have a headache or a period – you simply don't feel in the mood. What do you say and do?

As your old self: _____

_____

_____

_____

As your new assertive self: _____

_____

_____

Situation 4
You are in a social situation with a few friends. One of them brings up a controversial subject on which you have strong opinions. It soon becomes clear that your opinions are in a minority of one. It is obvious that they have not considered the topic from all sides. You have been patiently listening up to now. A friend asks you for your opinion. What do you say and do?

As your old self: _____

_____

_____

_____

As your new assertive self: _____

_____

_____

_____

Situation 5
You are looking forward to this evening. You have planned a night in, perhaps a nice relaxing bath, favourite TV programme, book, or whatever. You need to have a relaxing evening because tomorrow is a big day.

The telephone rings. It is Mandy, an old friend of yours. She says that she fancies a night out. She is feeling a bit miserable and wants cheering up. You guess that she has tried all her other friends and that they have said no. If she was a friend in real need you would willingly help her, but Mandy is always in a bit of a state and nights out with her usually end after 2 a.m. So you don't want to go out. What do you say and do when Mandy pleads with you to come out?

As your old self: _____

_____

_____

_____

As your new assertive self: _____

_____

_____

_____

Situation 6
Your husband/partner comes home with a surprise for you. He has
invited a couple of friends over for dinner this evening. You like the
friends, but you have now been landed with a dinner to cook without
enough food in the house, and you had been planning to spend the
evening on your favourite hobby. He has done this before and
promised to always ask you in the future. You are justifiably angry.
What do you say and do?

As your old self: _____

_____

_____

_____

As your new assertive self: _____

_____

_____

_____

To make sure that you are on the right path, here are some possible
assertive answers to situations 1–6. There is no one right answer. As
long as your answer sticks to the basic assertive principle, you are
doing fine.

1 You say something like this: 'I wonder if you could help me. I
   don't have a phone and with this delay my family will be worried
   about me. Would it be possible to use your phone to make a quick
   call to them?'

2 You interrupt the conversation by raising your hand, palm facing
   your friend, then say in a firm voice, 'I didn't realize the time. I

have to go to the shops right now, before they close.' You break eye contact and start walking towards the door, perhaps putting your arm through hers and gently taking her with you.

3 In a caring voice say, 'It seems that you would like to make love, is that right? I don't really feel like it tonight. Perhaps tomorrow, when I have more energy. Could we just hold each other before we go to sleep? I do love you . . .'

4 Speak out confidently, using all the knowledge you have to put your case across. State your opinions and try to make your friends see your point of view. See the issue from their point of view, too, and ask them to explain why they hold their opinions.

5 Don't let yourself go out. You will not be able to control the situation. To her pleadings, simply keep restating the fact that you do not want to go out. If she appears really desperate, you could compensate and ask her round to your house on the strict understanding that you will go to bed at 11 p.m. (and stick to it).

6 You tell your husband that you are angry with him. You could give him the choice of cancelling the evening or going out to buy the food and cooking it himself.

Conclusions to assertiveness

If you truly value yourself, you will stand up for your rights. The more you stand up for your rights, the more self-esteem you will gain. And having more self-esteem means you value yourself more.

This is a positive feedback circle, and makes a welcome change from those negative vicious circles that we met earlier.

The more your confidence grows, the more you will get out of life. You will attract positive emotions and dispel negative emotions.

EXERCISE

Self-assessment

Answer the following questions:

1 If you were consistently assertive, how would your eating habits improve?

2 Why would they improve? See if you can think of five areas for improvement.

Eating habits that would improve	Why would these habits improve?
1	
2	
3	
4	
5	

If your eating problem has emotional causes, being assertive will help resolve it. To accelerate the satisfaction of your emotional needs, the next section directly addresses those needs.

GETTING YOUR EMOTIONAL NEEDS MET

In Part 2 you may have identified that sometimes you eat in order to overcome some difficult or painful emotion. Being assertive usually helps by allowing you to take more control and power into your hands. You can take even more control over your life when you are clear about what emotional needs you have. This section will encourage you to be proactive in understanding and seeking your emotional needs. It is far better to know that you are acting to satisfy your emotional needs than to be simply reacting to emotional difficulties as they arise. In order for your eating/weight problems to be permanently solved, you will have to be emotionally robust to overcome life's challenges that will inevitably come.

Emotional needs, like any need, act as prime motivating forces. Once you have satisfied a need, you will not be motivated to get more of it. For example, if you are thirsty, you will be motivated to drink. When you have drunk enough, your motivation to drink more is zero. Your motivation will rise again as you become thirsty again. You obviously have many physical needs which operate like that. You will probably not be content if you have any physical need which is not being satisfied. In fact, the word 'satisfied' can be defined as having one's needs met. Emotional needs are just the same. You will not be truly content unless you have a degree of fulfilment to your emotional needs. So the big questions are: what are our emotional needs and how do we satisfy them?

Emotional needs

The aim of having our emotional needs met is to find happiness and avoid pain. Anything you do can be ultimately explained by these two instinctive drives. If we are not happy inside ourselves, it is very common to look for outside things to give us pleasure and take away the pain. It may be wanting a lot of money, perhaps wishing for a Lottery win to magically transform your life. It may be a promotion that will give you extra status. It may be new clothes, a new car, a baby, a new relationship or, of course, food. However, we all know, deep down, that if we take our unhappiness, our insecurities and our angst into a new relationship, a new job or even Lottery millions, we will still not feel happy on the inside, even though we could look great from the outside. There are many outwardly 'successful' people who are deeply unhappy inside. They often end up in a spiral of spending more on 'toys', taking more drink or drugs, more sex, more relationships – desperately hoping that the next thing will bring them peace. However,

The real cause of unhappiness is the lack of joy in our heart

Whatever external conditions we find ourselves in, it is what is in our hearts that counts. Darkness is only the absence of light. So it is the lack of positive feelings that allows the negative ones to dominate.

The eight heart desires

Every individual will have a different recipe for happiness. John Gray describes these in his book *How to Get What You Want – and Want What You Have* (Vermillion 2001). All happiness recipes will draw on the following eight ingredients:

1 Love and support from parents.
2 Love, support and fun from friends and family.
3 Love, support and recognition from our peer group.
4 Love and support from our intimate relationship.
5 Loving and nurturing ourselves.
6 Loving and supporting someone who is dependent on us.
7 Giving back to and supporting the community.
8 Connecting to a spiritual aspect of ourselves.

By looking at the above list, you may instinctively be able to pick out the emotional needs in which you have some lack. You will simply know that you are not satisfied in those areas. Perhaps there are items on the list that contain no wants, because you have what you need in those areas. Since we all have different needs, everybody has a unique path to happiness. That path is also constantly changing as life's events unfold. For example, if you enter a new relationship and everything is wonderful, it is very easy to neglect your friends. But after a while, when the honeymoon period is over, you suddenly realize that you haven't been in contact with friends, and you then feel a need to reconnect with them. That takes the pressure off your intimate relationship to satisfy all your emotional needs, and your relationship with your lover will improve. Also, what made you happy last year may not make you happy this year. So by constantly asking yourself: 'What emotional needs do I need to satisfy?' you will be keeping yourself on track for happiness. Before you answer that question, let us examine more closely the eight emotional needs one by one.

1 Love and support from parents
As mentioned earlier in the book, our emotional health was configured at an early age by the relationship we had with our parents. If your parents did not give you the unconditional love and support that you needed, is all lost? Thankfully not. The past can be healed, and as adults we need to make sure that we have gone

through that healing process. You may have to see them in a new light by really understanding why they did not give you what you needed. Were they themselves emotionally damaged by their own childhood? Were they misguided by working too hard to provide for you materially, and neglecting your emotional needs? By understanding them and their lives, it is possible for you to forgive and let go of any resentment or anger. In fact, it is essential for you to forgive. Forgiveness and compassion will set them and you free. Whether they are alive and by forgiving them your relationship will improve in the future, or whether they are dead and it is a matter of redefining your memory of them, it is very important to go through this healing process.

You may want to see a counsellor or therapist to help you through this process. They will give you the unconditional support that perhaps your parents could not give you. By understanding and forgiving your parents, many of the negative self-beliefs that they unwittingly imposed on you will be released. The maturity that comes from this forgiveness will enable you to parent yourself.

2 Love, support and fun from friends and family

This emotional need is about having a good time, laughing and having shared experiences with those who are close to you. Do you have enough of these times at the moment? Do you have good friends you can speak openly with? Do you have friends who support you?

If you don't, you may need to cultivate old friendships and develop new ones. Perhaps you need to spend more time with brothers and sisters and develop a closer relationship with them. Developing new friends is sometimes difficult. Just how do you break into a new circle of friends and meet like-minded people? It is especially difficult if career moves have meant that you have not stayed in one place for any length of time. Probably the best way is to join some club or society that engages in something you are very interested in. I joined a t'ai chi class and met a wonderful person who has become my best friend, not to mention three other friends with whom I am in regular contact. What are your interests? Go to the local library and look up interest groups, look in the local paper or on the internet. Get out and meet people who are interested in the same things you are.

If you are never in one place long enough to make new friends, ask yourself if your lifestyle is really the one that you want. Perhaps it was when you were young, but things may have changed. Maybe you want to put roots down in one particular community. If you are happy with your mobile lifestyle, perhaps you could make more effort to stay in contact with old friends, if only by e-mail.

Real friends accept who we are, warts and all. That helps us accept ourselves.

3 Love, support and recognition from our peer group

Isn't it great to be loved and appreciated by colleagues? There is an overlap between this need and the need we have for close friends and family, but in the peer group it is more about 'feeling one of the gang'. By joining an interest or activity group as mentioned above you will feel one of the gang, and the bonus is that you may find one or two of that particular gang who become real friends.

Human beings are tribal animals. Do you have a tribe that you belong to and identify with? If you do, you will recognize that the tribe has many shared values and rituals that define it. If you are in the tribe, you are somebody. Perhaps your work provides you with a tribe, but only if interactions and relationships within that tribe give you strength. In the rat-race of today, there are few workplaces that give that sense of security. If your work gives you this, you are lucky! There are parents' groups, single parent groups, charitable or religious groups, sporting groups, self-help groups, and so on. What tribe could you join? Think about joining a tribe as you, rather than as a partnership. Let your outside interests enrich your love relationship. It will give you something which is yours and something interesting to share with your partner. Also, it can be healthy for partners in a relationship to have their own sex tribe. Most women like being with other women and most men like doing things with other men, as well as with each other. Are you a member of a tribe of women?

4 Love and support from our intimate relationship

This need is for someone special in our life, a person we can love, share with, grow, comfort and commit to, a person who thinks we are special and treats us accordingly. We want a person who is dependable and trustworthy. We want to have wonderful sex where we lose our separate identities in a blissful union. You could probably add another ten attributes that you would want in a partner. The characteristics we want do not make it easy to find the right person. These days, our expectations are very high and most people do not have enough time to cultivate their relationship. This means that there are a lot of pressures on relationships. You really have to work at your relationship.

If you are in a relationship now, is it fulfilling your needs? If not, you will need to improve the relationship in some way. It is usual for the woman in a relationship to instigate changes. Most men find it more difficult to start talking about problem areas. So the responsibility may be yours. I can think of no better way than reading *Men are from Mars and Women are from Venus* by John Gray (Thorsons 1993). Read it first to understand the differences between men and women, then read it with your partner. Make it as unthreatening as possible. Most men are fascinated by the book because they begin to understand a most mysterious subject that usually baffles them: women. Come to a mutual understanding of the situation. Explore the concepts of the book together. Understand each other better and agree that you both need to change.

When we don't have such a relationship most of us have a strong need to find one. There are exceptions. Some people may have all the fulfilment they need in another area. For example, a nun who devotes herself to God may find that what she gets from this spiritual connection transcends all the other needs. But most of us are not cut out for the monastic life, and we do want another person to share our life with and perhaps create a family as well.

If you do not have a close relationship and you know that this represents an important need in you, what can you do? This is not the book to give advice about finding the 'right' partner. There are other books you may like to read that concentrate on this issue and that may give you some useful tips. But I will give you one or two thoughts to be going on with.

First, don't try too hard. This just causes anxiety and stress. Instead, concentrate on getting your other needs satisfied. You will need to do this anyway. That will get you out and interacting with new people in the first place. Second, hold the intention in your mind that you want to meet the partner who will 'expand your magnificence' as a human being. Don't go with a shopping list of the type of person you want. That limits you to what you already know and you might then miss what could be under your nose. Rather, focus on what you want the relationship to be. Third, don't think that there is one 'right' person. There are many potentially 'right' people out there. It is a matter of first meeting someone with that potential, then discovering if it will grow into the relationship you want. That means you will probably have to go through the process that used to be called 'dating'. Make it a low-risk 'getting to know you' phase. Fourth, don't expect perfection. If you do, you will always be disappointed and never commit to anyone.

5 Loving and nurturing ourselves

This need is about giving yourself what you want. It is about doing things which you like, and not about doing things for others. A simple example would be having a pampering day that is organized around you. My partner calls these her 'tiara days'. She sleeps as long as she likes, then has a long bath with her favourite essential oils, carefully applies nail varnish, puts on a dress and sometimes even wears a tiara. She assures me the tiara is not a delusion of grandeur, but is symbolic to her that she is not going to go out. That's as much as I know. It is her day and I don't pry. I suppose she then does whatever she wants. If you are able to nurture yourself, you are demonstrating that you think you are worth it. Think about whether you want to go to a particular place, do a particular thing (it could be anything – hang-gliding, dancing, beauty treatment . . .) or you may like time with a good friend. What would give you a lovely warm feeling in your heart? These special days will need planning. Enjoy the planning of your day. Put the next 'tiara day' in your diary.

Of course, it is good to think of doing small self-nurturing things on a daily basis. This means planning some time every day just for you. If you had twenty minutes every day just for you, what would you do?

Embarking on this programme is a sign of you loving and nurturing yourself. You are doing it for you.

Do you have a need for more self-love and nurturing?

6 Loving and supporting someone who is dependent on us

This need is about being responsible for another. Being responsible gives us a feeling of worth. It makes us realize we are grown up. The trust we receive from another brings out the best in us. We live up to that trust and it confirms to us that we are the grander human being that we would like to be.

The obvious people who are dependent on us are children. If you have children you will probably know the feeling of unconditional love that flows through your heart when you see them sleeping. I use the sleeping example because, as a parent myself, I know how challenging children can be. When I see my son sleeping it reminds me how wonderful and beautiful he is. It reminds me of his total vulnerability when he was a baby. My heart goes out to him. It helps me remember the grander part of him, after the cheekiness, the moans and the wants. I feel good about myself as a dad.

If you don't have children, or they have left home, how do you receive this particular need? If you have grandchildren, you have a perfect opportunity to be responsible for another. Do you need to feel more responsible for them than you do? If so, consider longer periods with your grandchildren. How about overnight stays or taking them somewhere special? If you don't have children, what other living thing is totally reliant on you? It could be a pet, a garden or indoor plants. I made a pond in my garden and every day I check what is going on there. There are fish to feed, newts and beetles to watch, weed to be cleared and marginal plants to be tended. I have to nurture it and it gives me back a good feeling. Apart from children, what have you got to nurture? What have you got that needs you?

7 Giving back to and supporting the community

If there has been one huge change in most of our lives, it is a breakdown of local communities. Everything used to be linked to the local community in the past. It is our local tribe. Perhaps some of the old communities were stifling and dogmatic, but in their healthy form they are supportive and give us a sense of place and identity.

This need is about giving back to that which gave to us and supporting the local structures that make a positive impact in the area. We all would like to live in a community where there are good facilities, a sense of people pulling together and where children can be safe, all happening in a pleasant physical environment. If there is a strong sense of community you will get support when you have difficulties. Community spirit will move you to help a neighbour if, say, their house is flooded. The human being has a need to give for giving's sake. The community spirit is made up of individuals' spirits.

People who are active in their local community are often mature. It is very difficult to give regular time if you have a job and children. So please don't think I am saying you 'should' give back to the community. You may not be at that stage of your life. But if life seems a little empty, and you have plenty of time on your hands, perhaps satisfying this need could be very beneficial for you.

As most communities are now vulnerable, you could make a significant contribution to your community. There is voluntary work for a whole range of people in need, from young to old. It may be driving someone without a car to the shops, it could be campaigning to save the local library, or perhaps a fund is needed to upgrade the children's playground.

Do you have a need to give to your local community?

8 Connecting to a spiritual aspect of ourselves

This need is about wanting to feel part of a bigger whole. If you feel that there is more to life than the immediate physical existence, you have a sense of the spiritual. If you feel that life is meaningless, it is because you have not yet found that your life is part of a greater pattern. Even without becoming too metaphysical, from a scientific viewpoint we are all connected. Chaos theory suggests that a butterfly flapping its wings in Brazil is connected with the breeze in our garden. How you live your life will affect other people, other animals, other plants and the environment as a whole. You do make a difference. Think about this life-teeming beautiful blue planet in a solar system of inhospitable planets. We are lucky! We are given this fantastic gift of life, but we take it for granted and too often focus on the problems and the pains.

The people who appreciate life the most are often those who have had to look death in the face. By facing death, you realize how precious life is. Facing death has led many people to change their lives. When something special is about to be taken away from you, you see it in a new light. You see all the qualities. You see everything you would miss. You would do anything to keep it. This awareness can transform the way people lead their lives. It can radically change their priorities in life. It asks the question, 'What is really important in my life?'

If you have a need to make a connection to something bigger than yourself, give yourself time to learn meditation or prayer. Mix with other people who are seeking a spiritual connection. When you are going through a crisis, ask for help 'from a higher source'. Even if you don't believe in God, you can receive strength and comfort by 'acting as if' there is something out there that loves and cares for you.

When you have your spiritual connection need met you will feel at peace. You will not fear death. You will not be needy. Then you will be able to overflow with love and compassion for others.

EXERCISE

Self-assessment

To what extent are your eight heart desires satisfied? Fill in the table below. Put down a figure between 0 and 10, with 0 indicating that no needs are met in that area and 10 that all your needs are met.

Heart desire	Score
1 Love and support from parents	
2 Love, support and fun from friends and family	
3 Love, support and recognition from our peer group	
4 Love and support from our intimate relationship	
5 Loving and nurturing ourselves	
6 Loving and supporting someone who is dependent on us	
7 Giving back to and supporting the community	
8 Connecting to a spiritual aspect of ourselves	

Your self-assessment will form the basis of your plan of action in Part 4.

Lifestyle and stress

With awareness of what our emotional needs are, it is hardly surprising that in our frantic modern society it is difficult to create a life for ourselves that truly satisfies us. Most people feel under some sort of stress. It is difficult not to. If you work, it is likely that your employer asks a lot from you. If you have children, they want a lot from you. If you have to travel some distance to work, that takes a lot out of you. If you have to juggle your money to pay the bills, that puts pressure on you. If you live far from your family, not having support makes you feel that you have to carry all the burdens on your shoulders. Sorry if I have depressed you, but that is what I see happening in our society. I think a lot of people are doing their best to carry on while feeling quiet desperation inside. I have yet to meet anyone who has a job who says that they have enough time to do everything that their life demands.

When we feel stressed, we start thinking and feeling differently. We think about surviving the short term, getting over the immediate problem. We have less patience with ourselves and others. Our immune system is weakened and we are open to infection. Our muscles tighten, particularly in our back, neck and shoulders. We find it difficult to be soft and loving. We may take out our frustrations on those closest to us, damaging the very relationships that we need to sustain us. In that condition, do we really care what we eat? Do we think how our bodies will be in five or ten years' time? Do we have time to satisfy our deepest emotional needs? No, no and no.

So why not take this opportunity to really think about your life and your lifestyle? Contemplate the following:

If you were on your deathbed, looking back at your life, what would you have wished you had done more of, and what would you wish you had done less of?

I would have liked to have done

More of in my life	Less of in my life

So why wait until it is too late?

Most big changes in people's lives mean giving something up. To have your heart desires fulfilled, you may have to give something up. If the cup is already overflowing, there is no room for anything new to flow into it. Deciding on what is really important in life and what is just an illusion or a distraction is probably the most important question in this book. Think about it and talk to supportive friends. You will discover that you are not the only one finding life a struggle. Be open to hearing about how other people have got more out of life by embarking on big lifestyle changes. But remember, you are unique. Don't just follow what other people have done; it may not work for you. Think about what you want, and how that can be balanced with your loved ones. Don't live life out of habit. Be bold and dare to create your life the way you want it.

CHANGING HABITS

If your eating/weight problem has no emotional factors, this section will help by guiding you through the process of changing habits. Even if there are emotional factors involved, you may have also got into some poor eating habits. So I recommend that everyone goes through this section.

Changing habits is largely about motivation. You need to be more motivated to adopt the new habit than keep the old one. There are two main motivators: the forward pull of moving towards something that gives you pleasure and the push away from something that causes you pain. If you make the pleasure of doing something new so strong and the pain associated with doing the old thing also strong, then pull and push are in the same direction. The new behaviour will become compelling. If we can make good eating habits utterly compelling, we will have solved your eating problem. But how do we know what are good eating habits? Although I promised you no diets in this book, it is important to say something about the foods we should eat.

The right foods

Of course, there are no right foods and wrong foods. It is simply that we should eat more of some sorts of foods and less of others. Here are some of the most recent ideas about foods:

- High carbohydrate consumption seems to satisfy the appetite more than high fat intake.
- Overweight people tend to have more fat in their diet than slim people.
- High carbohydrate foods include bread, potatoes, rice and pasta.

From the above, we can conclude that high fat intake is the big problem. High fat foods do not satisfy for long, but they do add a large amount of calories. After a high fat food, your body may crave carbohydrate because the body breaks down carbohydrate into simple sugars for energy. So after eating fatty food you may feel a craving for something sweet! That is obviously bad news. It would be the double whammy. However, if you eat a lot of carbohydrate you will feel more satisfied for longer. Carbohydrate is much bulkier than fat, so you can fill up.

We all know that sugar is described as empty calories and if you ladle it on your cereal or drink a litre of fizzy drink a day, you will be overdoing it. But sugar in marmalade, jam or desserts, in moderation, is not going to do much harm, and more importantly you won't be depriving yourself of the sweet taste. If you eat bulky carbohydrate as your main food, you will probably be content with sugar in moderation.

Carbohydrates have formed the basis of the diet of most civilized cultures down the centuries. Rice is the staple for most of Asia. Oats, barley and wheat were staples in Europe, millet in Africa, quinoa and potatoes in South America. As long as you don't have a high fat sauce with the carbohydrate, or have a huge amount of butter with your baked potato, you should be able to eat well and lose weight. When eating a dish like chilli con carne, eat more rice at the beginning than the meat sauce. If you are full up, it is better to leave the meat sauce rather than the rice.

Don't forget the pulses: lentils, peas, beans (baked, broad, chick peas, black eye, butter, aduki, etc.). These are nutritious foods with medium levels of protein. They are bulky and will fill you up. They have also been staple foods over the centuries.

Contrary to popular belief, the body does not need much protein. Cheese, meat, eggs, nuts and seeds do provide protein and minerals, but we only need a small amount each day.

Fruit and vegetables are, as we all know, the foods we should eat more of. Eat as much as you can of a wide variety. Fruit can be eaten any time as a snack, and vegetables will accompany your carbohydrate-based main meals. Salads, like fruit, are alive foods with plenty of vitamins.

Red meat is best eaten in moderation as it has a high fat content and takes a long time to digest. Be aware of all the high calorie food and drink that we often like to consume on a daily basis; alcohol, fizzy drinks, biscuits, cakes, cheese, crisps, peanuts, ice cream, etc. You don't need to stop consuming anything: simply be satisfied with a smaller quantity. Make it a treat which you enjoy. I like chocolate. My favourite is the 70 per cent cocoa organic dark chocolate. I buy it for a treat and may have two small squares after a meal. Because I eat without guilt, I can really savour them.

Convenience is a big factor these days when it comes to food and cooking. You have to make it easy for yourself (and maybe your family too). Pasta is very easy. Rice is easy (when you know how – learn if you don't know). Porridge is easy for breakfast (three minutes in a microwave). Potatoes are easy and versatile.

If you are not a soup-maker, I suggest you seek out a cookery book and get a few soups under your belt (as it were). The wonderful thing about soups is that with a handful of lentils or a few potatoes, a stock cube and any other vegetables, you have a tasty wholesome meal. If you eat meat, throw the bones in. Make a big pot every few days. Add some leftovers and it will change day by day. If all you have to do is heat up a pan of soup, slice bread and open a packet of salad for a great meal, cooking will not be a chore. The best kitchen tool I ever bought was a hand blender for £12 that you lower into soups to give them a whizz – and you just rinse it under the tap. Get a recipe for chicken soup, the great healing food from the Jewish tradition. That's a comfort food that really does us good.

Summary

- Make your main meals based on carbohydrate with vegetables (meat optional).
- Have salad with most meals. The vitamins are high in uncooked food.
- Eat regular meals so you will have less need for grabbing high fat fast food (e.g. crisps).
- Cut down on fried and fatty foods (including pastry).
- Have a small sugary snack if needed (*a* piece of chocolate is OK).
- Always have fruit in the house.

- Learn to cook a variety of soups and have a pot on the go all the time.

You will find cookery books that will give you some great recipes based on carbohydrate meals.

Now let's start work on your motivation. We'll begin with clarifying the pain associated with staying with your existing habits.

I've had it

Make a list of everything around food – eating, emotions, appearance, clothes, etc. – that you've had it with. What are you totally fed up with? For example, you might say, 'I am totally fed up with having to squeeze into my jeans,' or 'I am totally fed up with feeling shame and guilt about what I eat,' or 'I am totally fed up with feeling embarrassed about my body.' Use your own words and your own heart-felt examples:

_____

_____

_____

_____

_____

_____

Making a new neuro-mental association

Now you must link all the above list with eating the high fat foods you need to reduce. You are going to make a new NMA, which will direct the subconscious mind.

Picture in your mind a high fat, high calorie food that you want to cut out of your diet. Now around that picture see all the 'I've had its' in the above list. *Do it now.* You have to visualize the pictures to make this work. See in your mind's eye that particular food being associated with all the things that you are utterly fed up with. Use your imagination. *Do it now.*

When you've done that with one particular food, do the same exercise with another food. See the 'had its' in bright clear focus.

Surround the food with the things that you've had it with. Make the association very strong between the foods that you no longer want to consume and what you are totally fed up with.

Do this for all the foods you no longer want to consume. Of course, you may not want to cut out these foods completely, but simply reduce them. This exercise will help you do this, because the visualization is like putting a danger warning in your mind on to certain foods. They are available to you, but in small amounts.

Repetition and emotional intensity are the keys to success

Repeat this exercise regularly and make sure there is very strong negative emotion associated with those foods that you know you want to cut out.

Short term versus long term

One of the reasons we have to do the above exercise is because of the time difference between eating the wrong way and the negative results. If the moment you ate a cream bun, you saw another fold of flesh appear, my guess is that you wouldn't eat the bun. The problem is that food and drink can give instant gratification, while the 'had its' take longer to show. So that's why the previous exercise is designed to link certain foods to their longer-term effects. There is another NMA that will help.

Eating less NMA – re-educating the stomach/brain

We are often attracted to foods because of the way they look and how they will taste. In our natural habitat of hunter gatherers, we could eat whatever we could find. This was because we did not have many sweet things available, and the fat from animals was not a problem because our lifestyles would have meant we burnt up almost double the calories that the average person now uses. These days, we have infinite availability of high calorie foods, so we have to be more aware of what we put into our mouths.

We have to learn to listen more to our stomachs and bodies than to our taste buds. Too often we eat a high calorie food we like (particularly high fat food), and then feel lethargic and bloated afterwards. For example, eating pizza might be enjoyable, but if you eat until you are completely full, all that fatty cheese may make you feel slow and bloated. If we listen to our bodies, we will probably stop eating before we consume too much.

Change your attention to how you are feeling in your body

In order to do this:

- Eat more slowly – allow the food to settle in the stomach while you are still eating.
- Take smaller initial portions – you won't then feel you must finish the plate.
- Stop eating for a minute during a meal.
- Don't watch television while you eat – if you are concentrating on visual images you will find it difficult to pay attention to how your body feels and you may miss the 'I'm full' message.

Notice how foods like fruit, salads and vegetables make you feel. Do you feel lighter with plenty of energy? Listen to your body.

Your awareness will, over time, create a new NMA. This will be your new habit. You will listen to your body and feed it with the quantity and quality of food that it needs.

EXERCISE

Visualization – positive NMA

Before you do this visualization, make a list of all the positive things that will happen in your life when you have solved your eating problems. Think how wonderful you will look, how wonderful you will feel, what wonderful things you will be doing, etc.:

_____

_____

_____

_____

_____

_____

Now picture yourself eating delicious, carbohydrate-based meals with plenty of attractive fresh vegetables. See yourself eating more slowly and really listening to your body. Then surround that picture with all the wonderful things you listed above. See the whole picture. *Do it now.*

The brighter you make the picture and the stronger the positive emotions you feel, the stronger you make the association. *See the picture again.*

PART 4
Action Plan

Introduction

By this stage you should know the cause of your eating/weight problem and know how to solve it. Simply knowing how to solve a problem does not guarantee the solution. This part guides you along the easiest paths to that solution.

Your action plan will be drawn up over ten weeks, ensuring progress is made step by step and the changes within you are gently integrated into your life. Each week you will concentrate on three areas:

1 being assertive;
2 getting emotional needs met;
3 forming healthy eating habits.

ASSERTIVENESS

Refer to your personal problem profile in the Assertiveness section on p. 63. Knowing the cause of your eating difficulties, decide which of these problems, when solved, will help remove that underlying cause.

If you feel that there is a vital area which is not covered in the problem profile, include this in your list. Choose ten situations in which you would like to be more assertive. Put the least important problem at the top of the list, working down the list in order of importance. Below is an example of such a list:

1 *Receiving compliments*: I feel embarrassed when people pay me compliments.
2 *Expressing justified displeasure*: I am scared of complaining about food in restaurants and service in shops.
3 (Not on the personal problem profile) *Apologizing* even when it is not my fault.
4 (Not on the personal problem profile) I never follow through the punishments to the children because of *guilt*.

5 *Expressing personal opinions*: in a group of people I am normally the quietest one.

6 *Making requests*: I don't ask the doctor for more information.

7 *Expressing liking, love and affection*: I don't tell my husband what turns me on sexually.

8 *Standing up for legitimate rights*: I let my mother boss me about as though I was still a child.

9 *Refusing requests*: I am unable to say 'no' to overtime.

10 *Expressing justified anger*: I bottle up my feelings, especially anger over my husband going to the pub too often. This makes me feel all burned up inside.

Write your priority list:

Assertiveness priority

1 _____ (least important)

2 _____

3 _____

4 _____

5 _____

6 _____

7 _____

8 _____

9 _____

10 _____ (most important)

You now have a list of ten situations in which you want to have more control and feel more confident. Now you can transform your list of problems into a list of goals. We do this by rewording the problem; below is the example list reworded into ten goals.

Priority goals

1 I will say 'thank you, that is very nice of you' when I receive a compliment. (*I do have many qualities and it is good when someone appreciates me.*)

2 I will politely let the waiter know if there is something wrong with the meal, rather than muttering under my breath that I will never come to the restaurant again. (*I am the customer and I have a right to comment; my views will help improve the restaurant.*)

3 I will stop saying 'sorry' all the time. I will stop saying 'sorry, it's only me' when I ring my husband at work; instead, I will simply say, 'It's Jane.' (*I am as important as anyone else.*)

4 I will not let my child's sulking make me feel guilty. I will stick to what I know is right. (*If he knows I mean what I say, he will respect me and our relationship will improve.*)

5 I will share my opinions and ideas with others. (*My opinions and ideas have a right to be heard. They are important to me and they deserve to be respected.*)

6 I will ask the doctor to explain in more detail anything I don't understand. (*After all, it is my body and I take ultimate responsibility for it.*)

7 I will start telling my husband what turns me on sexually: 'I'd really like it if you did . . . , that's really nice . . . , what would you like?' (*I want to be open and honest with my husband, I deserve to ask for what gives me pleasure.*)

8 I will make it clear to my mother that I can make my own decisions and take the consequences, although I will still appreciate her opinion. (*It is high time that my mother and I formed an adult to adult relationship. I am grown up.*)

9 I will politely but firmly refuse overtime when I don't want to work the extra hours. (*I want to be in charge of how I organize my life.*)

10 I will express my feelings and emotions at the appropriate time and I will let my husband know that I am angry about his boozy nights. (*If I feel justified anger it is better to express it rather than suppress it. It is another way I am being honest and authentic.*)

Goals and beliefs

Before you write your list, it is important to understand how the problem list was reworded to become the list of goals. Goals are positive statements of action. They say what you will do, rather than what you won't do. Goals state the solution, not just the problem. *This rewording is very important. It directs the subconscious.*

In the above list there is a statement in italics after each goal.

These statements represent beliefs, which are as important as the goal itself. You need to develop underlying positive beliefs about yourself which become the bedrock of your actions. *You must believe in why you are doing something for it to work.* When you write your list, add the underlying belief that empowers that goal, as I have done in the above example.

Now write down your priority goals by rewording your assertiveness priority list. Your top priority goal will be at position no. 10 on the list, because it represents your biggest challenge. Your lowest priority goal will be at position no. 1.

Priority goals (with underlying positive beliefs)

1 _____

2 _____

3 _____

4 _____

5 _____

6 _____

7 _____

8 _____

9 _____

10 _____

ACTION PLAN
Goal fantasy

You now have your assertiveness goals listed in order of priority. Before you begin this fantasy, go back to your goals and spend a few moments thinking about each one. Next, read through the fantasy and then actually visualize it in detail.

EXERCISE

You are walking down the street and see an old-fashioned blue police box ... Your curiosity makes you peek inside ... it's unbelievable ... it's Dr Who's Tardis, his time machine. The instructions are simple and you set the dials to six months into the future. You want to see how life will have changed for you when you have achieved your ten goals. You decide for a six-month jump ahead, because that will have given time for people's resistance to your changes to disappear and their respect for you to grow.

Take a deep breath and press the button. A strange whistling noise ... flashing lights ... then stillness ... The electronic calendar shows the Tardis has taken you six months into the future. You can now ask the Tardis computer to show you pictures of yourself as you have become, on a big TV screen ... It's incredible, you are looking at how you wish to be. See the screen showing you the new you in each of the ten problem areas, one after the other. See yourself having achieved your goals, now performing with ease and confidence in all the ten situations.

What is your body size on the screen? If you like your size, that's fine, you have chosen the right goals to solve your eating problems.

If you don't like your size, go back into the fantasy and change your size to one which you do like ... See yourself performing as well with this different body size ...

If you cannot see yourself at your desired body size, even with the changes made in your assertive behaviour, now add in your eight heart desires, your emotional needs. Imagine all your emotional needs are fully satisfied. Now go through the fantasy again. How are you looking and feeling as you watch yourself on the screen in six months' time?

Before you start the next section, be sure your goals are the ones that you feel are right.

You may want to revisit the beginning of the programme and work through the sections again. Many people discover new things when they approach the same material for a second time. There are concepts presented in this programme that take time to fully understand. When you read a book or watch a film for the second time, it is amazing how much you have missed first time round. It may also help just to observe what emotional factors affect your eating, before you finally decide on your priority goals.

HOW TO ACHIEVE YOUR GOALS

Your goals will be achieved when your conscious and subconscious minds are working together. Your subconscious is rather like a car, in that it is powerful but it has to be driven in a particular direction. You have to give your subconscious regular and clear-cut commands. It can be somewhat stubborn and often needs a push in the right direction. But once it has a clear indication of what you want it to do, you'll be astonished how it will work for you. It takes the struggle out of success.

Because you now have well-defined goals
you can give well-defined commands

In order to build a pattern of success it is very important to start with the most easily achievable goal and work progressively through to the hardest goal. This is based on the principle contained in these two proverbs: 'Don't jump in at the deep end' and 'Learn to walk before you run'. The best way to motivate yourself is through desire and success. The stronger you desire to achieve your goals the more likely you are to succeed. That success will motivate you further as your confidence grows and you enjoy all the good feelings that naturally follow.

So you are going to start Week 1 of the ten-week programme with Goal 1, the least important goal. By concentrating your mind on one goal at a time, the goal should be achieved comprehensively. Also, by starting with the least important goal you will feel freer to experiment and make mistakes, which are all part of the learning process. As you work through the next ten weeks achieving one goal

per week, by the time you reach your more important goals you will
be enjoying positive reinforcement from earlier success.

As well as assertiveness goals, you will include actions to satisfy
your eight heart desires. Let's now look at the heart desires again:

1 Love and support from parents.
2 Love, support and fun from friends and family.
3 Love, support and recognition from our peer group.
4 Love and support from our intimate relationship.
5 Loving and nurturing ourselves.
6 Loving and supporting someone who is dependent on us.
7 Giving back to and supporting the community.
8 Connecting to a spiritual aspect of ourselves.

Looking at the above list, which of the heart desires need most
attention? Which ones need filling the most? Think about the impact
on you and your life of having each need met in turn.

Now make a priority list for your emotional needs. Unlike your
assertiveness priorities, put the heart desire that is in most need of
satisfaction at the top of the list. The reason for this is that it can take
some time for your actions to bear fruit. So start with the heart desire
that will have the biggest positive impact for you. Refer back to the
section where they are explained in detail (p. 72).

Heart desire priority

1 _____ top priority

2 _____

3 _____

4 _____

5 _____

6 _____

7 _____

8 _____

DIRECTING THE SUBCONSCIOUS

This section is vital to your success. It is one thing to know, but another thing to do. It is virtually useless to read this section without putting the principles into practice.

Practise the following exercises with each goal in turn throughout the coming weeks. So if this is Week 1, it will be Goal 1 that you are working on.

Weekly affirmation cards

Get ten blank pieces of card. Write Week 1 through to Week 10 in the top corner of each card. Next, write down each assertiveness goal in bold letters on each piece of card. Then add the underlying belief underneath it. Finally, add the action you are going to take in order to get your heart desire met. This last part is best added as you start each new week because it is difficult to predict what progress you will make.

There is no reason why you can't progress more than one heart desire at a time. There may be a logical sequence of stages. For example, you may have to book your 'tiara day' now, and also find out about local interest groups, or start meditating.

In our example, Goal 1 concerned receiving compliments with ease. If the heart desire in most need of a boost is love, support and fun from friends, and if it is the fun part that is particularly missing, the affirmation card would look something like this:

Week 1

Goal: I will say 'thank you, that is very nice of you' when I receive a compliment.

Belief: I do have many qualities and it is good when someone appreciates me.

Heart desire action: Ring up Marge and ask her if she would come with me for a weekend in Amsterdam.

Carry the current week's affirmation card everywhere with you. Look at it regularly throughout the day. It is your special helper. Love, support and nurture yourself. It will keep you focused on what you have to do. *Take the first step.*

Visualization

There are three visualizations to help you with each goal each week. To gain access to deeper levels of your subconscious – because this is what visualization does – it is beneficial to create the right atmosphere:

- Do any chores first, so they do not nag on your mind.
- Find a relaxed few minutes, free of interruptions. Disconnect the phone.
- If you find it difficult to relax, do something first that helps you unwind (e.g. have a hot bath, do some stretching exercises, or listen to relaxing music).
- Prepare yourself by taking five deep, slow breaths, inhaling through the nose and exhaling with a deep sigh through the mouth, saying the word 'relax'.
- Sit upright in a chair with your hands resting in your lap, palms facing up. Relax the shoulders.
- Close the eyes.
- Say out loud, 'I ask for infinite love and healing to come into my heart now.' Repeat this out loud at least ten times.
- Continue to say, 'I ask for infinite love and healing to come into my heart now' in your mind for as long as you like.

You should now be feeling more balanced and peaceful. Move on to the visualizations when you are ready.

> ## *EXERCISE*

Visualization 1: Goal achievement – to be done every day

1 Spend a few minutes running through the whole scene as though your goal of the week has been achieved. Fill in as much as possible, everything that is said and done ... How is your self-esteem affected?

2 When you feel comfortable with running this basic scene in your mind, introduce difficulties from the other person(s) involved. Make them try to resist your assertive behaviour ... See yourself coping with them without getting uptight, but keeping cool and in control.

Practise these visualizations until they become so strong that you really expect them to become reality. Remember, *your beliefs are your reality.*

Visualizations 2 and 3: Food and body – to be done every day

1 Picture yourself with food, being just how you want to be around food. See yourself enjoying good food and eating slowly ... Imagine you are now satisfied, having eaten only a moderate amount ... You are listening to your body signals and take delight in finishing eating when you are satisfied ... and you have energy ...
2 See yourself with a body shape which is realistic and acceptable to you ... Enjoy how you look ... not just the body shape, but your glow of health and happiness.

Visualize on the bus, train, etc.

As well as at prepared times, try visualizing in different places. We often daydream when looking out of the window, on a bus, in a car. If you have been having a difficult time in your life it is easy for negative thoughts to arise when you are daydreaming. Remember, darkness is the absence of light, so bring light to your mind by visualizing your goals.

What if you can't visualize?

If you find visualization difficult, it doesn't matter too much because it is only one part of the goal-achieving strategy; spend more time affirming your goals out loud.

THE REAL-LIFE SITUATION

The energy that you put into self-knowledge, understanding the principles of assertiveness, satisfying your emotional needs, the affirmation cards and the visualizations, will pay handsome dividends when you come to the real-life situation itself. Here are some extra tips:

- *Stage nerves*
  Some of the new behaviour patterns may produce a little anxiety, which is normal when you do anything new. Any actor will tell you that some adrenaline boosts their performance. You may feel like an actor initially and then you and your role will merge, to produce a balanced confident person.
- *Mistakes are OK*
  Don't worry about making mistakes and not being perfect from the start. Learn from your mistakes. *Mistakes are an opportunity to learn.* Build up so much desire to change that difficulties will not stop you from succeeding.
- *Laugh*
  In this serious business leave room for humour. You will know that you are progressing when you can laugh at yourself. When being assertive, a smile goes a long way.

FINAL WORDS

Well, you've made it this far – well done!

Virtually all my clients who put this programme's ideas into action achieved what they wanted in terms of weight and eating. What they didn't know at first was that they were going to enhance virtually every aspect of their lives at the same time. I hope that you will be equally surprised and delighted.

You will have to re-read the programme a few times to obtain a full understanding of the ideas presented. Use it as a reference manual to help you achieve each goal.

You are embarking on a ten-week action plan, but many people see it as part of longer-term personal growth and development. It may take months and years to fully integrate new ways of feeling and behaving into your life. Enjoy the process of change and growth. Love yourself and love others.

APPENDIX
Ten-Week Planner

You need ten weekly charts to complete during the programme. Take this book to a photocopy bureau and ask them to enlarge the following chart to A4 size. Get ten copies, one for each week. Update the chart every evening while events and feelings are still fresh in your mind. If you need more space, attach a separate sheet. At the end of the week, fill in the heart desire and the self-esteem boxes.

GOOD LUCK!

Week No ....   Date ....

Visualizations	Sun	Mon	Tues	Wed	Thurs	Fri	Sat
Affirmations							

Tick above boxes when completed each day

Changes in my eating habits

H
e
a
r
t

d
e
s
i
r
e

Fully met

Half met

Not met

Changes in my feelings and behaviour

Emotional
needs met
(fill in the tube at
end of week)

I'm great

I'm yuk

Self-esteem
(fill in the tube at
end of week)

What I like about myself

Flashes of self-knowledge

Any other thoughts or messages to myself

Assertiveness goal of the week_____

Action this week to satisfy emotional needs_____